heart broke

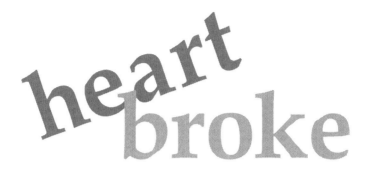

from uncertainty to possibility
(how I learned to trust in truth)

Christine K. Monaghan

Published by Wild Pearl Storytellers, West Vancouver, BC, Canada
© 2010 by Christine K. Monaghan
Printed in Canada and the United States of America

All rights reserved. No part of this publication may be reproduced or transmitted in any form or by any means, electronic or mechanical, including photocopying, recording, or by any information storage and retrieval system, without the prior written permission from the publisher or the author. Contact the publisher for information on foreign rights.

ISBN: 978-1-4538-9174-2

Edited by Brenda Judy
www.publishersplanet.com

Cover Design by Amanda Merrifield, Paul Nash and Harrison Brown

Interior Design by Carolyn Sheltraw
www.csheltraw.com

Cover Photo courtesy of Amanda Merrifield

∞ The paper used in this publication meets the minimum requirements of the American National Standard for Information sciences - Permanence of Paper for Printed Library Materials, ANSI Z39.48-1992.

www.healthmentorship.com

in memory of Debrah Rafel

I dedicate these words to *Wild Pearl*, my dear pal, Debrah Rafel. She initially encouraged that I come to know my voice within through the written word, by journaling. Her nudging inspired my listening to the voice within, the one I now refer to as vitalheart. *Wild Pearl* introduced me to the immeasurable gift of silence during her weekly yoga classes. She passed away recently during the prime of her life from a superbug, and left behind twin baby girls and her newlywed husband.

Our time together the last three years was infrequent, but she was and always remains an amazing imprint in my life. She demonstrated gentle strength, possessed a graceful stance, was strikingly beautiful and ultra feminine with always a dash of aqua blue. Her demeanor was strong as an ox, though delicate in appearance. Each time I begin my regime with yoga DVD in hand, I whisper, "Hi." I know you're smirking as you witness my own gentle transformation. Your life was cut short, and yet, you remain in essence.

One day over tea, we dreamed up the term *Wild Pearls*, denoting women who are rooted in their individuality, graceful in demeanor, and possess enough wild spice to actualize their unique potential and beauty, internally and externally. You, my dear, are the poster woman for *Wild Pearls*. This written accomplishment is my gift to your legacy, the power of your spirited influence in so many *Wild Pearls*.

contents

Preface ix
Acknowledgements xi
Chapter 1: The Crumble 1
Chapter 2: Trust in Truth 15
Chapter 3: Heart*B*roke 23
Chapter 4: Fire in the Belly 45
Chapter 5: Yin & Yang, the Balancing Act 67
Chapter 6: Owning Your Potential 87
Chapter 7: What You Resist Persists 101
Chapter 8: Intuition, the Vitalheart Voice 111
Chapter 9: P.S. I Love You 129
Chapter 10: Uncertainty & the Global Heart 143
www.healthmentorship.com 163
Give-Back and Collaborative Partners 165

preface

So, why *From Uncertainty to Possibility?* The notion of transforming uncertainty into possibilities is relatively new to me in terms of being consciously aware of it pervading my daily existence. My relationship with uncertainty was certainly more fear based than love based up until five years ago.

For as long as I can remember, my method in dealing with uncertain circumstances was to *make something happen*. This would externally nix the perceived unpleasant circumstances and, internally, quiet my anxious, worrying chatter. I became proficient in *making it happen*. However, fear was running this show as the external fix more often than not delayed addressing an internal strife. Of equal importance, in the pursuit to eliminate the associated yicky feelings lickedy-split, I missed many new possibilities by rushing to find a fix. So, the process for internal growth, peace and healing was abruptly stalled.

For years, I lived this way until my *crumble* five years ago. The time had come to stop dousing uncomfortable feelings, to learn to really trust in truth, and to regenerate my depleted, exhausted self from running away instead of befriending a great ally—uncertainty.

These writings represent five years of living and learning to trust in truth through choosing to view uncertainty with fresh eyes and an open heart.

The more I trust in my truth and lead from this place, the more frequently I experience new possibilities that otherwise may not have occurred, or would have taken years to naturally present themselves if I'd been in push mode.

acknowledgements

I have immense gratitude for all those who championed my efforts during this process. It has been an extremely humbling period that served me well with plenty of rich insights.

A great thanks to all the contributors to the book who took the time, energy and heart to share what their trust in truth perspective is in relation to a specific chapter with you, the reader: Cheryl Brewster, Christine Brown, Silken Laumann, Dr. Lee Pulos, Mirabel Palmer-Elliott, Ruth Stern and Fawn Christenson. Thanks to all my weekend editor friends, who invested their precious time, love and individuality into reading a chapter and providing me candid feedback: Mum, Dad, Lee, Gordo, Ron, Tweets, Bet, Cheryl, Marcia, David, Jeanie, Jenn and Bob McKay. RayC Moon, thanks for keeping me laughing with the e-mail jokes.

Much gratitude goes to Mary Reynolds-Thompson, the founder of Write the Damn Book. Your bi-weekly tele-coaching sessions were invaluable to my becoming a so-to-speak writer. I cherished the fun, spirit, trust and truth that you, Jenn and I shared. Astrid—Thank you for your loyal friendship over the years. You have been such a big fan of mine and I am of you as well. Sally Shields, you're the bomb! You are such a demonstration of grace in action. Thanks for truly showing me how to serve others first, with love, respect and purpose.

I'm amazed by the brilliance of youth. Amanda Merrifield shot the front cover image at age 14. You, teen miss, have unlimited potential if you choose to trust in your sense of self and purpose. I'm a big fan of what your possibilities are! Harrison Brown worked on the cover design with Amanda in between swims at the beach across the street. Harrison, you have a creative flare that will flourish with time and commitment. Paul, you were able to take Amanda and Harrison's creation and polish it for publication. I thank you for making Amanda and Harrison's talent shine!

CL, your enthusiasm, grace and *in-my-face guidance* when this work was at the publishers and required one more observant, knowing eye from the heart is my blessing. Our kinship nurtured throughout the years is a rare one with bouts of hysterical laughs and much in-the-moment shared silliness.

My sweetie, thank you for the gift of time, space and your quiet, powerful love. It provided me the sacred environment to get creative and do this. I'm wowed by your ability to demonstrate living in the now. You are my gem.

Lastly, I want to acknowledge Carol and Ian. You were there for me when my world crumbled. You literally and figuratively saved my life. Your individual and collective demonstration of love is rare and truthful in the context of being unconditional. Anyone who is fortunate enough to have you in their world is blessed, and is already very certain of this fact. I wish you as much abundance as you both so freely extend to others. Your lives are rich beyond measure in experience, thought and with those who surround you with their love. I love you both dearly.

chapter 1
the crumble

PRE-CRUMBLE DAY, THURSDAY

I'm off to a prospective investor meeting to reel in a cool million cash injection to grow my company. It's another frenetic day and there is no end in sight with deadlines galore. A dear pal is along for the ride, my extra set of ears and eyes as I feel very off, not trusting myself. I haven't been on my game for two weeks. Today, I feel super odd, but chock it up to mounting financial fatigue and PMS cramps. The last year, a series of hard straight hits to the ground has taken its tolls in ways I have yet to comprehend.

It's hard to shake off the internal, incessant debate to reschedule the meeting. I try to ignore the persistent weird physical sensations plus the utter exhaustion that washes over me. I push forward, not trusting the internal pleading to simply stop and rest. My justification is that maybe this meeting will shift the chaotic, stressful madness of my life toward a return to a healthy routine of ease. This financial investment will cure depletions on numerous levels.

The investor meeting is successful despite my rushing everyone. I feel off, with an out-of-body anxiety. The investor consensus is utmost confidence to provide funding for what they believe is a unique and timely business model. My business, a national seminar series program, educates individuals to own their potential through presentations delivered by leading experts in the financial, spiritual, emotional, physical and intellectual realms.

Post meeting, two girl pals and I head off for some retail therapy to Babalicious, an underground intimate wear shop. I am convinced that money and fun can be had in hosting home parties for silky sweet nothings and sex toys. In hindsight, I realize this as the diversion it was . . . there was far too much on my plate with the business and training for a half-marathon race. The latter of the two isn't such a stretch given my 42-year young athletic bod is in mighty fine form.

Dinner time arrives and I finish a spicy tuna roll and half bottle of Granville Island beer while watching TV with housemates, Carol, Ian and the two dogs. We have become extended family over the years, sharing plenty of ups and downs along with fabulous laughs and entertaining dinner parties. Lifelong bonds have been forged. I sip my beer and realize Rudi, my chocolate Lab, hasn't been fed. I make my way downstairs to the cupboard to get her food. When I step up onto the hall rug, I experience a wave of tired dizziness like never before. Everything is swirling. I fumble to sit down on the well-heeled Persian rug, which wafts doggie aroma from daily tromping, but the attempt is futile.

My next recollection is acute awareness of soaking in utter bliss—a state of sensational dreaminess not experienced before. It feels like a luxurious body cream concoction of bliss, peace and lightness being sensually massaged over every inch of me. I find it surreal witnessing myself in this state while, at the same time, being fully cognizant of not being conscious. My internal chatter beckons me to just pull out of this state, but a resistance pulls me further down, drowning in the bliss. The feeling is so polarized from how I felt all day, and, in hindsight, the last year.

My analogy of the heavenly state is being enveloped in the ultimate orgasmic sleep. Then, a sharp disruptive flash within my head competes for my attention. I literally try to shake off the loudest tone-ring blasting within my head. I'm aware of existing in two dimensions, the orgasmic blissful state and the other, a pragmatic survivor pushing through whatever it is that is happening to me at the moment. The masculine and feminine energies are battling for dominance.

"Call 911."

"No, don't call, Carol. I am fine." I snap back into reality as the masculine, pragmatic survivor rallies.

"Call 911. Chris, wake up," Carol pleads. Her words now compete for attention with my orgasmic state.

"Don't call 911." I'm back out of the orgasmic sleep again. My vision goes from blurry to in focus with Carol kneeling next to me and Ian standing above.

"Don't call 911; I am okay. It must be my period." I demand authoritatively, trying to regain control in this very out-of-control situation.

After what feels like moments to gather my wits, though much longer, I prop up on my side and am violently ill. Next, I'm sucking ice cubes, which taste like Bollinger's finest. Ian checks my pulse. It is too faint and low and I sense concern by all.

"My blood pressure is always low . . . always has been . . . no worries." I reassure us all.

By shifting into my *make-it-happen* mode, I intend to rewrite this destined happening. During the next wave of nausea, throwing up and killer period cramps, my honed negotiating skills deny what is occurring. I convince all three of us it is a vile flu. So, I buy myself another 16 hours or so on the living room couch; at which time I come to know what truly sick feels like, drifting in and out of a semiconscious state.

CRUMBLE DAY, OCTOBER 1ST

My dizziness and passing out returns with increased vigor and frequency. The Doc observes me coming to after passing out while seated on the toilet. He stands frozen at the bathroom door. A few weeks prior, I'd scheduled a checkup with this doctor as I felt so tired and dizzy when training for the half marathon. His advice then was not to worry, it was just stress. Now, I was headed to the ER.

Carol asks me of the Doc's whereabouts. I shrug while pulling my disheveled self off the toilet to prepare for the ambulance arrival. I try brushing off being abandoned by the Doc, without as much as a check of my pulse.

It's true, firemen are delicious specimens. They arrive with the paramedics. I'm outfitted with an oxygen mask and blood pressure band for the hospital-bound ride. I'm aware that something fairly serious is transpiring when drilled with questions between bouts of passing out. Out the back window, the stunning fall day whizzes by. I soak in the gorgeous, green stately trees and vivid bronze leaves falling through the stellar blue sky as I think what a perfect day for a run. Everything is surreal as the reality sets in that a run today is probably out of the question.

All sense of time is skewed as I get wheeled into an emergency room after repeatedly passing out and coming to on the stretcher in the lobby area. A human-sized plastic spatula is slid behind my back, which lifts me from stretcher to bed as I initiate hoisting myself over. I fiercely hold onto normalcy in this attempt, doing it on my own. My ignorance is bliss and a diversion that serves me well in this moment.

Next, I'm sporting more wires and an IV, though I wasn't conscious for their placement. I can't imagine what all the commotion is about, for what I'm trusting is simply menstrual symptoms or a flu ailment. I'm my own observer as my calm mind and eyes casually wander from this machine to that, as though watching boats sail by from a porch couch on a lazy summer afternoon. But, there are subtle, deliberate focuses on the EKG machine—beep, beep, beep. Who's to say what I scan for, but scanning I do more frequently than a calm individual would. I suppose I'm watching for suspicious activity—as if I will know what that looks like.

I come to, again, with oodles of activity whirling around me. Numerous staff are hustling, conferring and doing god knows what. I have no choice but to surrender to *what is*. Both arms now sport blood pressure bands, which squeeze so tightly my hands tingle. I voluntarily rub the healthy pregnant doctor's belly as she fires me with questions about medications or alcohol consumed today. I choke up with emotion, wondering how two healthy, vibrant women can be experiencing such dualities of health at this moment. I fight to stay in the room with her without understanding what the fight is about.

The nurse, Rob, wraps a pre-warmed blanket over my legs and tummy as I shake uncontrollably. Days later I understand it was shock setting in. With my eyes closed, the beep, beep, beep barely silences the guttural moans of a woman coming off her overdose in the next cubicle. Though neither charming nor reassuring, ironically, I wonder how one gets so distraught with life as to purposely try to end it while another fights to stay alive when circumstances suggest a premature and abrupt end.

Only a few thoughts stand out during this period of time in the ER: Chrissie, grow your hair long and curly again; Chrissie, take the rest of the year off, maybe until February if you want; Chrissie, close the business; and, Chrissie, write a book of columns based on the ones written for the seminar series newsletter.

* * * * * * * * * * *

Hi ho, hi ho, off to the OR I go! With gown on and nail polish removed just like an ER episode, my two girl pals, who have been in the ER with me since arrival, exchange silent smiles with me, which mask our fear. Sisterhood solidarity runs deep and, though we're all freaking out internally, we go with the perfected, strong, nonchalant façade. Somewhere in the mix, I believe I offend the on-call cardiologist by sourcing a second opinion through my pal's dad, who is a surgeon.

"You don't like me do you?" he utters from my bedside.

"I don't know you to like you or not, I'm just making sure this is the right choice given the type of surgery planned with such urgency in the next half hour," I respond.

"I can't do this without you Christine. You need to figure out how to stay." Laura's words are firm, a mix of reprimand and dictatorship.

So, I dig deep to retrieve a quiet power. My only request is that Laura stays overnight in the hospital, in my bed next to me. She stays. And, the nurse repeatedly boots her out to sleep in the visitors area when she returns to snuggle up with me.

The OR is clinical, overly bright, cold and uninviting. I'm wheeled through the back corridors with a portable EKG machine and heart sparker in case my heart decides to stop beating. I'm en route to the 45-minute, pacemaker implant surgery. Isn't this what happens to elder people with weak hearts? I just ran the half marathon route a few days ago! What the . . . ! I'm the healthy, athletic one in our circle of friends.

My naturally low blood pressure combined with an athletic prone low blood pressure plus a short in my heart's electrical system is causing my blood pressure to plummet, resulting in my passing out. Bradycardia is the medical term for this condition. I am sedated, so I'm not anxious, but aware of everything. The routine procedure involves a two- to three-inch incision in your chest just below the collar bone, above the heart. The pacemaker gets tucked onto the muscle with wire leads connecting the pacemaker to the ventricle and atrium. It regulates the rhythm as needed. For me, the $25,000 titanium gadget will spark when my blood pressure falls below 60; otherwise, my healthy heart continues serving me beyond its first 42 years.

My OR recollections are simultaneously sketchy and yet vivid in Technicolor. Time stands still, yet, certain moments stand out; I lie still, stark naked; I feel a haunting cold, noticing the portable EKG machine by my side; I indulge appreciation in my very decent, in-shape 42-year-old bod; I wonder if surgeons and staff simply see a slab of human flesh needing mending or if acknowledgement of a well-honed female body crosses their mind for a nanosecond—how do they filter human instinct out of the equation?; I engage eye contact with the young, handsome surgeon—an unspoken dialogue conveys my trust in a collective, non-negotiable healing energy to pull me through. Our eyes lock momentarily, then he detaches with an ingrained, trained response as he preps for his role.

The anesthesiologist introduces himself; the portly nurse is sweet and attentive. I look at the large tent-like sheet that is erected just below my neck. At first, the room lighting is overly bright, then dim. I lose track of what takes place next. Then . . .

I witness them working on me over there, somewhere to my left, though I'm not sure where I am. Who is this person observing me per se from afar yet within me? Once again, I reside in two dimensions.

"You need to get back over there, Chrissie." A voice within dictates me to move over to them while I observe them working on me. Then . . .

"Feeling a bit dizzy right now," I say to the nurse, regaining consciousness from another realm.

"I would imagine so my dear, your heart just stopped four times in a row. Good thing you are in such great shape," the nurse replies casually. She is kind and her stature somehow provides me comfort.

* * * * * * * * * *

POST-OP

Simple pleasures are sublime. I'm in good company with the post-op nurses Patti and Kim. They are attentive as I enjoy a little water and throat lozenge, which soothes my charred glass-like sore throat, probably from the throat tube. I recall and share my recent visit to a psychic. The psychic told me of a major health event happening, but not to fuss as I'd be fine. Until this very moment, I'd forgotten and blown it off as ridiculous, woo woo stuff. After all, I'm in excellent shape, eat super healthy, sleep plenty, drink only socially and don't smoke.

POST-CRUMBLE SATURDAY

What the hell just happened? I never saw this one coming as I return home 16 hours later with a pacemaker implanted in my young chest. I have no intention of sleeping solo as vulnerability and surrender to *what is* settles in. I feel a shattered trust, which goes way beyond betrayal for what my consummate athletic body has just endured.

Arrhythmia is a medical term that refers to a heart rate that is outside the normal range (60 to 100 beats per minute). An arrhythmia that is too slow is called a Brady arrhythmia or bradycardia, where the beats are less than 60 per minute. This is my condition. I remember going for a run last week and thinking my heart rate monitor wasn't working as it registered 40. That run was interrupted as I felt like all energy was draining out of me into the pavement, so I turned around and walked home before going out to a Jack Johnson concert later that night.

Sleep becomes my most frightening time of day. George Winston's instrumental calm serenades me. Ian and Robin give me nightly massages to George in the first week post-surgery hoping this relaxing diversion will shift my attention off the thudding pacemaker. Ironically, this gadget should represent comfort, but is a constant reminder that it remains the only thing standing between life and death for me. I'm officially dependant on a something . . . not a someone, but a something. What the . . . ! To this day, I rarely sleep on my left side as I feel it tick tock away, though I'm grateful and feel blessed for its place in my heart.

POST CRUMBLE SUNDAY
I sip mid-morning tea at the dining table with Laura and Carol. We discuss a sleepover schedule until my sense of safety and confidence returns to sleep solo. Our adrenaline high of the last few days has digressed into utter emotional and physical exhaustion. Carol and Laura need to get back to their routine and families.

The pacemaker sleepover list is done. A call is placed to my recent romantic interest. He returns the call a week later, promising lunch the following Tuesday, which never takes place. He is the first one of more than I like to admit who doesn't show up so to speak. It is a painful, lonely process but a necessary evil to once and for all be truthful for what I want my inner circle to look and feel like. The sleeping buddy schedule begins a weeding-out process for who my true friends are. It is the first of many pivotal learnings to confront truth and truly build my trust by accepting *what is* in uncertainty.

. . . .

Back-to-back, life-altering, romantic, health, financial and spiritual experiences over a three-month period resulted in what I now refer to as *the crumble*. I transformed my relationship with innate trust, which quietly nudges me toward a feel-good state as the norm, not the exception.

Since *the crumble,* I've embarked on a self-imposed, impassioned learning curve to discover the art in living my truth by trusting. I witness that the more truth lived, the more my life effortlessly unfolds in magical ways not initially envisioned. Now, more often than not, I feel rooted in the present, yet am aware of a well-paced momentum. I'm finally equally landed in body and spirit in ways strived for daily, but fell short of, for years. I'm practicing the art of letting life unfold. For ages, I understood the premise of letting go but never connected with how to recognize or feel its presence.

For me, learning to trust has been in questioning where my truth resides from the mundane to the complex. I've questioned mundane habits such as carrying protein bars and nibbles of food in my purse to life impacting decisions such as the ideal romantic partner. I've dissected who I was at 17, 24, 38 and, now, at 42. I believe trust begins in the now by defining current truths. A driving force is: What if time runs out and I don't get it right? My heart now springs wide open with compassionate candor and simple acceptance for *what is,* no matter how mucky things get. In turn, tidbits of trust are born.

With baby steps toward a sense of safety and certainty in both the certain and uncertain, I begin to revisit my relationship with uncertainty given it permeates every part of my present existence. A renewed vitality in my step will eventually prevail once I accept and trust in uncertainty.

Many mantras are dreamed up during *the crumble.* The first was created to make decisions on the basis of whether my choice will get me closer to or farther away from a refreshed ideal. If closer, I go forward; if farther away, it's a no go. At first, this approach is extremely black and white, but it is eliminating the stuff dragging me down. My one consideration is making sure I never intentionally set out to negatively impact another in the process.

My life story to date is comprised of equal parts: messy, chaotic challenges, and blissful, thriving experiences. *The crumble* is the catalyst for me to commit to a life of truth that is productive and purposeful to the best of my conscious ability. It has humbled me as I uncover my purpose in this lifetime. My purpose is to help others source possibilities within their uncertainty by trusting in the vitalheart voice, their intuition.

These writings are my perspectives in *the crumble* aftermath. These perspectives emerged from the depths of self-pity, poverty, loss of passion and absence of purpose—an overall sense of lack. In navigating unchartered terrain, these perspectives encouraged me to travel with fear's fury and come out thriving with ease and acceptance in abundance. If just one individual absorbs these perspectives and, as a result, ups the ante in living their potential by trusting in their truth, then my purpose is fulfilled. Now, that's vital!

> ♡ A man who becomes conscious of the responsibility he bears toward a human being who affectionately waits for him, or to an unfinished work, will never be able to throw away his life. He knows the "why" for his existence, and will be able to bear almost any "how."
> — Victor Frankl

connect possibilities
body · mind · spirit · heart

INTERNET RESEARCH

Cardiac Electrophysiology . . . . www.wikipedia.org/wiki
Cardiac_electrophysiology

Heart Block . . . . www.hrspatients.org

Heart Library . . . . www.heartlibrary.com

St. Jude Pacemaker . . . . www.sjm.com

Web MD . . . . www.webmd.com

MUSIC

David Gray . . . . www.davidgray.com

Dido . . . . www.dido.com

Norah Jones . . . . www.norahjones.com

READ

In the Meantime by Iyanla Vasant . . . . . . www.amazon.com

The Places That Scare You
by Pema Chodron . . .www.Shambhala.com/pemachodron

chapter 2
trust in truth

♡ Say not I have found the truth, but rather, I have found a truth.
— Kahlil Gilbran, the Prophet

I get it now. I know that to live my raw, unfiltered version of *a* truth is to allow trust to direct my way. I've coined the term *Vitalheart* to express this perspective—the inextricable voice of wisdom connecting trust and truth, my innate intuition.

On October 1, five years ago, my world as I knew it changed. I now aptly refer to the circumstances prior to and after this date as the *crumble*. HeartBroke articulates my general perspective of *the crumble* on a physical, emotional, financial, spiritual, romantic and intellectual level.

I don't intend to convey *how to* steps for what you *should* or *shouldn't* do to understand or live in relationship with truth. This would be arrogant and indicate that I really haven't learned my lessons from *the crumble*. Trust and truth are universally different for each individual based on beliefs, experiences and feelings that form an individual's perspective. My primary goal is to provoke your exploration of the trust in truth concept. If, by reading these writings, you identify what your ideal experience can be, what you will feel, who you can become when consciously living innate truth from a place of unwavering trust, then I'll feel ecstatic for the both of us.

In setting out to achieve this, a sharing of my experiences, others' perspectives, an array of resources and posed questions will assist you to ponder the trust in truth concept. Moment-to-moment choices truly demonstrate our level of trust in a given truth. In the end, it's your reflection, desire and interest in understanding what makes up your world within, your truths guided by trust in the vitalheart source—your innate intuition.

When referring to this perspective of trusting in truth, let's assume such universal truths as the ocean, the air we breathe, the stars in the sky, the sun and the moon. Agreeing on this assumption allows freedom to truly consider one's own interpretation of a given truth.

How do influences, environmental circumstances, present state-of-mind beliefs, feelings and experiences influence your current truth from the mundane to complex? How many of your thoughts, actions and beliefs are on autopilot? How are current or past experiences with love, family, career, friendships, health or religion impacting your truth? Do these truths actually belong to someone else who played an integral role in your life? What role does money, or lack thereof, play in what your truth is in respect to: what you purchase, what you believe is affordable, what you perceive your sense of worth to be in relation to your bank account balance? How do circumstances keep YOU stuck due to a lack versus abundance mentality—your perceived truth around the almighty buck? It's not about the money; it's all about the money! How about stirring up new possibilities by replacing exhaustive, destructive worry energy with *how can I create the next best thing?* Choose raising your good vibrations.

A question you may want to ask yourself is this. *Was I taught this way of truth or have I consciously determined this in my own highest good?* Then, decide how to best serve you and others to genuinely move forward with respect and grace. Don't underestimate the power and insights in questioning the mundane. Eventually, this automatically trains you to process the complex with ease. It becomes the foundation in sifting through significant decisions less the angst. What level of trust are you willing to invest in your most precious commodity, YOU? I believe this ultimate commitment to self can translate into optimum potential.

Truth isn't necessarily pretty when we come face to face with our creations of poor choices. The task is to switch focus off others and what they have done, or how they affect our circumstances, and place full responsibility on our self. By assuming all responsibility for what is or is not ideal, our truth speaks loud and clear. In stuffing down the real deal now, we merely delay it bubbling up at a later date.

Crisis and uncertainty is usually a catalyst, forcing our hand to face *a* truth. It rattles our senses to come to grips with that which is not serving us when we're figuratively dying in order to free the noose we placed around our own neck. If not respected, it can manifest into a Heart*B*roke bankruptcy in the form of a physical, emotional, financial, spiritual or intellectual dis-ease. If conscious enough, we heed this flag and evolve through worn out, mucky truth and onward with a vital, thriving heart once again.

The following vitalheart perspectives are shared by an array of individuals from various ages, income brackets and experiences. My thought is, the more fully you understand what others perceive *trusting in truth* to be, then, hopefully, the more inspired you are to truly think about the level of its importance to your vitality. My wish for you is a life that not only flows with ease, but thrives based on clarity of your truths and trust in this perspective, which frees space to flourish in ownership of your potential.

TRUST

♡ Firm belief that a person or thing may be relied upon, confident expectation, responsibility.
— Oxford Dictionary

♡ Letting go of a specific outcome or timing for a certain desire and allowing it to unfold in its own way and time, to be guided by ones intuition.
— Christine Monaghan

♡ Faith placed upon a person or occurrence where one believes that the intention behind an outcome will be carried out with integrity and honesty.
— Carol Lavery

♡ It is a lesson which all history teaches the wise, to put trust in ideas, and not in circumstances.
— Ralph Waldo Emerson 1803–1882, Essayist, Philosopher and Poet

- Trust is "the extent to which a person is confident in, and willing to act on the basis of, the words, actions, and decisions of another."

  — D.J. McAllister

- In her book, Barbara Misztal attempts to combine all notions of trust together. She points out three basic things that trust does in the lives of people: It makes social life predictable, it creates a sense of community and it makes it easier for people to work together.

  A critical element in studies of trust behavior is power. One who is in a position of dependence cannot be said to trust another in a moral sense, but can be defined as trusting another in the strictest behavioral sense. Trusting another party when one is compelled to do so is sometimes called reliance, to indicate that the belief in benevolence and competence may be absent, while the behaviors are present. Others refer only to coercion.

  —James Coleman

· · · · · · · · · · · ·

TRUTH

- Quality or state of being true.

  — Oxford Dictionary

- Choosing to represent who you have become today versus whom you were yesterday, last week, last year or 20 years ago. To lead this way without judgment or criticism of another, and with utter trust and grace in you. To honor that inner voice that quietly whispers or harshly screams to your physical self, the vitalheart source.

— Christine Monaghan

♡ What you believe is the nearest to being the real thing . . . the real essence or spirit of an idea or story. And their link? You cannot have trust without truth. Trusting relationships need to be based on honest feelings and honest communication.

— Carter Helliwell

♡ When a woman tells the truth she is creating the possibility for more truth around her.

— Adrienne Rich

♡ There is nothing to fear except the persistent refusal to find out the truth, the persistent refusal to analyze the causes of happenings.

— Dorothy Thompson

♡ All truths are easy to understand once they are discovered; the point is to discover them.

— Galileo

♡ If you tell the truth, you don't have to remember anything.

— Mark Twain

♡ Truth always rests with the minority, and the minority is always stronger than the majority, because the minority is generally formed by those who really have an opinion, while the strength of a majority is illusory, formed by the gangs who have no opinion—and who, therefore, in the next instant (when it is evident that the minority is the stronger) assume its opinion . . . while Truth again reverts to a new minority.
— Soren Kierkegaard

♡ If you do not tell the truth about yourself, you cannot tell it about other people.
— Virginia Woolfe

♡ The world is too dangerous for anything but truth and too small for anything but love.
— William Sloane Coffin

♡ But Whose Truth is the True Truth?

With enough attention to anything, the essence of what you have been giving thought to will eventually become a physical manifestation. And, then as others observe your physical manifestation, through their attention to it, they will help it to expand. And, then, in time, this manifestation, whether it is one that is wanted or not, is called "Truth."
— Excerpt from *Ask and It is Given: Learning to Manifest Your Desires* by Esther and Jerry Hicks (Teachings of Abraham)

chapter 3
heartbroke

I am Heart*B*roke. The particles of my once robust, healthy heart now represent losses over time in numerous shapes and sizes. An immense loss exists where previously assumed optimum, physical strength and health was the norm. Grieving a recent romantic loss makes my heart ache for what could have been if timing were on our side. It's amazing how abrupt the loss of passion for business is within my heart. A heaviness of spirit absorbs a loss of youthful innocence, assumed health, fun, verve and silliness. Seriousness for *what is* settles into my very being.

My truth—I'm at a complete loss of how to begin to trust in just one part of this broken self again. It is overwhelming and the idea of snuggling under my duvet covers indefinitely feels decadent, lavish and well-deserved under the circumstances. Moments of peace and ease have been lost to fear, uncertainty and sadness.

Heart surgery has sparked so many firsts. I believe the many firsts will eventually mend the shattered particles of my spirit, so it can brilliantly sparkle again, bit by bit.

I'm engulfed in uncertainty. It's pervasive in my breath, which is ragged instead of fluid, absent of a steady rhythm, similar to my heartbeat. *The crumble* is providing the opportunity to come face to face with my Heart*B*roke state. This emotional bankruptcy stems from events pre- and post-heart surgery. Future possibilities exist in acknowledging the many subtle and not so subtle untruths, which reveal themselves as *firsts*.

These firsts transcend worn-out daily routines, beliefs and behaviors and reawaken my eyes and consciously paced heart. It's time to take responsibility for veering off course and initiate resuscitation and forgiveness to repair this bankrupt soul. This process ends up taking the better part of five years to fully integrate the many new ways in leading. I'm fascinated to witness such shifts in perspective when conversing with others. Catching up to these firsts and their core impact on how I now live will take a lifetime.

> ♡ Nobody has ever measured, not even poets, how much a heart can hold.
>
> — Zelda Fitzgerald

. . . .

OCTOBER, WEEK ONE

There are firsts galore: my first bath as I feel invalid-like and move slow and shaky; my first cardiology appointment prompts anxiety; my first time navigating with the right hand as I'm a south paw; my first experience feeling emotionally wrecked; my first time surrendering to *what is* with not an ounce of push left; my first experience of acute sensitivity to light and sound; my first experience in dealing with a severely whacked-out nervous system, resulting in no appetite; my first time being concerned in looking skinny—it's an unhealthy, trauma-based leanness of the loins . . . an atypical female response.

Over the following five weeks, my routine is simplified. I need help getting into and out of the tub as my left arm movement is limited until the pacemaker settles in. The chest bandages need to stay clean and dry. Vanity is alive and well, which I take as a good sign by asking for help with body shaving upkeep. Yes, it's a feeble attempt to fill the dry, emotional well. Navigating with my right versus left hand isn't working, so mascara, tampons, bra and anything beyond hair goop are nixed from the equation. My wardrobe consists of several two-piece Lululemon workout ensembles with zipped hoodies. This provides ease for moving my left arm in and out of clothes. I enjoy the freedom in the newly forced, temporary habits. It simplifies things and dulls the sting of overwhelm and pressure.

Wild, irrational thoughts of reaching too high and the pacemaker leads snapping inside are a constant source of irrational terror associated with moving my left arm. I fight to abate this fear taking hold. It is exhaustive, which further weakens my body and spirit. My former *push* mode is giving way to a quiet, innate determination to build a new, healthy normalcy in lifestyle.

Waiting to be called at the cardiologist's office seems like an eternity. I gaze at the mostly elderly patients as I admire another stunning fall day through the window. Why am *I* here in this shaky, vulnerable state when, just this time last week, I ran 18k in between negotiating a million dollar investor? Can I really have been taken out so quickly by such an event? All sense of safety eludes me. The nurse's closet-type office barely holds two comfortably with no ventilation. I request the door remain ajar to alleviate the humid, claustrophobic wave hitting me. Fidgeting with my Tiffany's bracelet provides a diversion and subtle reminder of terrific successes. I'd spoiled myself with this purchase when I successfully carried out the seminar series tour in two cities. It symbolizes an outcome of my strength, perseverance and empowerment through clarity of vision.

Finally, my first cardiologist appointment is concluded. A complete health inventory finishes in moments with nothing noteworthy revealed and no medications to review or to prescribe. My inquiry if burping is normal is confirmed with more oxygen now circulating within. This translates into air bubbles trapped in my stomach. A lamented medical card will arrive by mail to carry with me. My chest bandages can be removed in ten days and a stress test appointment is set for six weeks. I will come for annual checkups and can never undergo an MRI, ever. With that, I'm sent on my merry way to life as it was . . .

Calls from Tweets, our family nickname for my younger brother, proves a daily source of encouragement to me. In addition to other sporadic well wishers, his calls in particular continue long past when the masses get on with their life during week two. His voice holds less fear as time passes. His daily check-in begins with a 1–10 rating. I fudge the notches up a bit to combat his fear as much as mine. His calls mean more than he may ever understand and always end with, "*You are an amazing woman, Chrissie, and I love you.*" Some days, I hang onto his words as though he's sitting next to me, they prod me forward. This encouragement reminds me of the many amazing experiences to date. I tell myself that one day I will see *the crumble* in this light as well. There is plenty of amazing moments still ahead of me.

Gorgeous aromatic flowers arrive. Fresh batches of chicken soup and another Lululemon lounge lizard outfit brings a pick-me-up to the days.

I clock in for beddie-bye time about 7:30 p.m. as the dark shadow of sleep appears. Early to bed is the norm as dizziness and emotional exhaustion prevail from coping in self-driven chaos the last week and, probably, the last few years. Sleep is my enemy, tamed marginally by the soothing sounds of George Winston and Enya. I try to sleep. I lie still and feel the loud tick tock in my chest as Robin, my dear friend and Thai masseuse, treats me to a weekly candlelight massage. I create a sleep mantra, "I will not pass out anymore as I am covered with the pacemaker, and am safe and in optimum health."

My friendship with Robin is cemented. Our intimate conversations expose complete trust by sharing our respective truths, a vital aspect in healing. Sleeping buddies come and go. If not for fighting with my internal mad chatter, it might feel like fun, childhood sleepovers where giggles and magical memories are made.

Two separate spa treatments are sweetly arranged by women pals. One would assume this to be a relaxed proposition and just what the doctor ordered. But no, I'm on high alert. Arriving for the facial, I scan the machines to try to identify which may possibly interfere with my gadget. I arrive home exhausted. The well-meaning pedicure treat isn't anymore peaceful as intuition shouts *no* to the vibrating massage chair. A subsequent call with the cardiologist confirms that the magnetic field in massage chairs interferes with titanium tickers.

Worry consumes me as I zoom through the retail store entrance detector just to be extra safe. One day I almost knocked a woman over who was at a standstill rummaging in her purse. Doesn't she know I can't stand idle in the middle of these sensors for God's sake? Enough already, Chris! But, new firsts just keep confronting me to shift from worn-out perspectives.

Fanatical describes my three times weekly vitamin shot at the Naturopath, intended to boost the healing process. Supposedly, it calms my very fragile, over-worked nervous system and adrenals. Desperation for relief from anxiety and worry fuels this obsession. Sleep is fitful and eludes me as I lie sideways with one pillow in front and another behind to mimic spooning and being spooned on my right side.

Brief hints and stints of residual confidence appear over a few weeks when I take my courage pills—trust. I insist it is time to sleep solo as dependency lurks close by. I organize my bath with the exception of help rinsing my hair, which I holler downstairs for Ian to come to the rescue. I take my longest walk to the end of the block and back four times. I eat smaller meals more often, so my blood sugar evens out. I surrender to an attention span of a six year old for reading or watching TV and, in turn, surpass my record of 12 rounds of solitaire in a single sitting. My only desire is to build strength back and create peace of mind. I've learned that human beings truly enjoy helping, they just need to be asked or given a reason.

* * * * * * * * * * * *

Tap, tap tap . . . the sound of romance knocks on my door. Tick, tick, tick . . . the feel of emotional bankruptcy beats in my heart. I am unnerved.

Male visitors come and go throughout week two of my recovery. Their presence causes me to reflect on romantic choices to date with not much else going on. I sense how far from my ideal I had flitted with my recent relationship.

I'm shut down for romance, but still contemplating romance's future role—how will he place, feel and live within my world? The thought of being physically intimate and entwined in pleasure with another scares me. Fear and uncertainty over my loss of sensuality and womanly appeal rattles within as I stand naked, in front of the mirror. I see only a protruding gadget under my collarbone. I wish for more fat on this body part for concealment purposes, a first asking for *more* fat. My otherwise quite perfect chest, neck and collarbone area now marred with the protruding gadget. Damn it anyways, why did I push so hard for so long?

My conviction around no intimacy is put to the test way sooner than I could have imagined. A visitor of the male species, a once could-have-been lover, drops by. He sits close to me on the sofa. His masculine appeal and scent tweaks the once vibrant sparkle in my eyes. He prods me to reveal what lies beneath my chest bandage. With a quick rip of the bandage, a small, thin, three-inch incision sitting on top of a two-inch diameter oval is revealed—my pacemaker tucked just under the skin. Though swollen, I find it odd versus scary to see the protruding gadget. With a bit more fat on my bones, the victory scar and protrusion will hardly be noticeable. He half kids me about testing out the new gadget to see how it works. I resist anything more than hugs and a quick smack on the lips. Two years will pass before I'm ready to intimately connect again.

I enter a period of evaluating the best parts about various lovers to visualize the next *Mr. Right*. My most recent choice is a source of excruciating heartache, leaving me feeling shattered and ashamed for giving my heart to someone who couldn't fully reciprocate. The romance is indicative of bad judgment and being off kilter in the months prior to surgery. I'd sworn I'd never find myself in a situation like this one and, though I'd extracted myself from this unhealthy equation shortly after engaging in it, shame still sears my heart, smothering it in regret.

I decide that to have a remote chance of healing my bankrupt spirit and heart, I must come to grips with being solely responsible for what is or is not part of my circumstances. This is a chalky pill to chew, but one necessary to ensure I don't end up a bitter, twisted sister. So, I acknowledge the regret I hold for my recent romantic circumstance, forgiving myself in little bits, otherwise, the regret will short-change me of what I truly deserve in love. And, I choose to carry forward with me the love, inspiration and spontaneity shared from the best of the best male vintages to date.

Raw emotion stings sharply, tugging at my heartstrings now more often than not. Truth be told, this sting consumes its share of heart space over the next couple of years. Fantasy carries me through solitary, sleepless nights of struggle with dreams of a beloved holding me. He assures me I'm not alone, kisses my scar, and I feel sexy to him and to myself. He lends me his strength to navigate this unchartered territory, and then I awake, alone. This emotion wells up from deep within when in the presence of men and extends beyond romance, striking my core with the uncertainty prevalent in all areas of my crumbled world.

In the presence of men, I surrender to a new experience of acute physical and emotional vulnerability. My soul is depleted from giving. I'm uncomfortable and awkward with this newfound exposure. I feel something strong, but what? The gadget is a slap in the face of my perceived pre-surgery health and strength. Relentless, self-recrimination for overextending my finances to increase viability just to be forced to contemplate bankruptcy haunts and eats away at me. Last summer,

I denied the flag of exhaustion and continued: pushing to level ten on the treadmill to experience *feel-good* endorphins; pushing to a new level of reckless, disrespectful outflow of energy with the naïve belief it would be reciprocated.

How is it that I've come to develop so much acumen and, yet, remain so naïve about unearned trust? The net outcome is emotional bankruptcy, which is proving to be the most difficult to recover from. This crumble will eventually draw me to the most precious of gifts—I must trust this as my truth, my gospel.

. . . .

A flag now, and in the months following, signals that I'm *doing* versus *being* more than is healthy when my head gets woozy and my appetite vanishes. No appetite is a first for sure. So, I respect the flag and surrender by pulling back in the moment of awareness as this gift presents itself. I realize how developed my masculine energy is from business and know the time to cultivate a softer, feminine way toward ease is here.

OCTOBER, WEEK TWO

I encounter more flags in the form of firsts this week, signaling a need for change. My first true meltdown and freak out arrives with a panicked telephone conversation to my psychologist friend. Home delivery of her customized CD promising cellular healing and serenity arrives at lightening speed. A sudden realization of the impending financial, physical and emotional fallout from the surgery is creating waves of panic, like restless bugs crawling just under my skin's surface. I acknowledge that I'm emotionally paralyzed with uncertainty and have no clue of how to begin to pick myself up.

I Google Post Traumatic Stress Disorder to decide if I need professional help—I opt for the CDs in the interim. As I listen to the CD three to four times daily for weeks, I tell myself to simply focus on making this hour peaceful. Each hour, the intent is to feel a tiny bit better than the last one. My state is fragile, fearful and needy. I loathe myself in this state and an innate survival fight to feel my way through this weakened, grief-stricken mindset is set in motion.

The waves of panic represent an internal truth that I'm no longer prepared to just make it happen anymore, but how do I deal then? This worn-out way, which has dictated and influenced my entire life for better or worse, was supposed to protect me against exactly this sort of situation. By this situation, I refer to not being able to fully take care of myself, to not feel fully strong in self, to be so vulnerable and fragile that a healthy, normal way of functioning is in question.

Being pissed about being in this situation, where I feel reliant and needy, is an understatement. I've spent my life creating independence for myself. The only way to blow through survival mode and thrive again is to learn to surrender to *what is*, hour by painful 60-minute long hour. I want my truth to be that I utilized all this muck to once and for all create solid ground by choosing awareness.

Healing tonics are uniquely packaged but consistent in delivery: my girls host a silver service, high-tea party complete with Kentucky Derby hats, crustless deviled egg sandwiches, home-baked oatmeal cookies—very civilized and delicious; my autonomous task of folding laundry and making the bed spells normalcy; my successful seven-block walk; my healthy restlessness to tidy the kitchen with one arm; my stance made with the web developer calling under the well-wishes guise, then cornering me on when his contract balance will be paid given my surgery—nice; my decision to pass up two projects given no mindset; my opportunity to say no to that which drains instead of adds energy; my commitment with the personal trainer arriving weekly at my doorstep for recovery workout, his treat; my honoring dizzy, wooziness as a flag for pushing too much—I obey like a besot lover; my *tick-tock* check-in call from my business partner, championing me for our pending investor meeting. He (Don) is among the few good choices this past year—an extraordinary individual of integrity.

My woozy moments are becoming a *trust in truth* opportunity. I'm learning to walk away SOONER from situations and people who demonstrate through their actions that my best interest isn't at heart. This means right away, instead of permitting excuses and justifications to muddy clear insights. Hanging in to fight the good fight isn't necessarily the best course of action as we've been lead to believe.

. . . .

OCTOBER, WEEK THREE

I start taking action in week three of recovery to diffuse mounting anger: I meet with the doc who left me on the toilet, he responds to the surgery by saying, "It is so weird." That's it for this quack—the next doctor would never dream of leaving my side should I be in need of an ambulance; I set off to the library with the ridiculous notion to gather information on writing a book for my column; I venture to the local soccer field with Rudi and Discman in tow to exercise—with a newly laminated pacemaker card tied to my shoelace; I run with tears streaming while listening to Christina Aguilera's *"Thank You for Making Me Much Stronger"*—I complete a 12-minute walk/run interval workout.

Getting angry is healthier than staying anxious. From the exterior, I'm another fit, healthy, well-healed West Vancouverite strolling through her daily errands. Internally, I fight to tame my raging madness. Constant questions are a call to action, to shift to a healthy place instead of this internal typhoon, which may drive me mad from exhaustion with what little energy presently remains.

With many tears of anguish, I feel pressured to course correct and soon, knowing that if I don't, I'm headed for an extremely dark place I'm not sure I can extricate from. So, one hour at a time, I consciously make choices to get me closer to, not farther away from the evolving ideal, a refreshed truth. *The why me* phase ends up serving me well as I: demand answers to my present circumstances, not as a victim, but from a pragmatic standpoint; demand searching arrhythmia, heart block, electrical shorts, pacemakers—Google becomes my ally as courage ekes me forward; demand truth of my financial position, getting real with what options are available. Overall, action lessens the sense of overwhelm on all fronts, if for no other reason than to trick the ego into believing forward momentum is happening.

Internal chatter and questions relentlessly skip from finances to romance, to physical well-being, to the future, to what ifs. This assures me I'm still engaged in life, prepared to commit learning the lessons to shift what's needed to experience peace, and resolve chaos once and for all. I will need to cultivate gentle patience, surrender to quiet and tap lots of love to truly receive the lessons. Once received, then utilizing them to productively and purposefully coexist in this world from here onward will bring ease.

My questions range from: "Who or what wounded my heart?" *to* "What is the pain within?"; "Why have I chosen to give more attention to others' needs than mine?" *to* "Is there fulfillment in any part of my life?"; "How do I navigate moving forward without being at a standstill?" *to* "How do I let go to effortlessly move forward without pushing?"; "How will I know when I've gained the lessons intended from this set of circumstances?" *to* "What will it feel like to live a life feeling at ease as the norm?"

OCTOBER, WEEK FOUR

My commitment to course correct continues. I feel like I'm on the witness stand throughout the investor meeting and the first ten minutes are blurred as waves of anxious dizziness dominate my attention. Somehow, I spew out the necessary dialogue like so many presentations before and calm returns with another internal mantra reassuring absolutely no obligation for me to direct anything to happen, or commitment to *do*.

I resolve to raise my energy, to eliminate tangled muck as new situations require this resolve; I eke out a giggle at the mall when a gym acquaintance ignorantly asks, *"Can you walk far with it?"*; I send an email to the seminar series presenters, notifying them the company is on hold and receive many nurturing responses; I heed words of caution "easy does it" from my brother flagging recently full days, *"Pace yourself, Chrissie"*; I enjoy an inspiring lunch with a dear friend from back East, planting seeds to co-create a woman's retreat, *"Easy does it, Chris"*; I love the sound of laptop keys tapping as I languish in the therapeutic journaling frenzy; I crank up the tunes to weed out waves of anxious dizziness and negative thoughts to complete another workout routine; I negotiate borrowing money from friends to cover a few months expenses; I indulge in the inspired love of drop-by visitors; I confirm an appointment with the trustee, assuming the close of my business; and I continually scratch my scar—it is healing quickly. Now, I need to do the same emotionally.

Beyond these tears, lies anger and forgiveness—an angel reading by a friend.

All these firsts are markers as to where various truths lie.

My spirit literally shifted in the moment I chose to leave the blissful, orgasmic altered state and return to life on the hall rug the day before heart surgery. Why was I blessed with this second chance with life? It creates a commitment to evolve with utmost accountability for my highest potential. In negotiating with the universe to live this commitment, I acknowledge my ultimate purpose is not yet discovered. This shift will require accountability to not screw with my precious being or others, and live authentically by trusting in my truth. Interestingly, previous therapy sessions uncovered the duality between my unhealthy sense of responsibility and its role as a terrific resource. Everything and everyone is up for reflection, not judgment, but rather inquisitiveness about what my truth is as I honor this second crack at life.

Confronting untruths is messy work, and, make no mistake, work I created all by myself consciously or otherwise. These revealed untruths can become the healing salve to many draining, internal and external wounds making up my current state of affairs. Enormous accountability weighs heavily. A certain manic energy to shake myself awake to gently trust truthfulness is replacing the "make it happen" ways of days gone by.

I am HeartBroke on many levels, yet the time has arrived to once and for all decide what life is to be and create it, period. I feel value for life in a manner I believe only happens when someone or something is taken away from you too soon, when it doesn't add up, and never will. My wish is to hold onto this urgency, to cease the preciousness in the ordinary daily activities.

Lead as you would like to follow based on your beliefs. I realize that to manifest the ideal, I need to walk this daily, then it will perpetuate a positive cycle for all concerned. I strive to live simplistically each day through clarity of my beliefs with the intention of leading from here. In practicing this way, more energy returns. I learn that in the past I kept busy so I didn't need to confront all that was not congruent for me. When super clear on my truth, I convey it with less judgment of others and concern where their truth rests. This is due to being rooted in mine for the right reasons, none of which are about anyone else. This practice is challenging.

Sometimes, intuition flags that I'm receiving selective information from another with pieces absent from the whole story, which aren't in my highest good. It becomes a test for trusting that my belief will eventually create freedom for all involved. I find myself in situations where standing alone isn't fun or comfortable in the moment, but without fail, a quiet power ensues when going with *what is* for me. Leading from this place cracks my world open to connect with like-minded trust in truth seekers, not for the faint of heart or approval pleasers, for sure.

I believe in speaking my truth in written or verbal form, it provokes a greater possibility for reciprocal, genuine dialogue. Recipients of my truth access more of who I am and, then, can choose to engage or not. It's transparency at its best and, hopefully, encourages a conveying of their truth. This is vital for me in relationships of any sort. I've ruffled a few feathers along the way by divulging my truth while the masses kept it zipped. I understand the hesitation to do so, but never wished leading otherwise in hindsight. For me, it's the most direct route to the next right place, even if unrest is experienced in the interim.

I also believe we certainly aren't intended to endure the challenges nor relish in ecstatic moments to settle into mediocrity and smallness of self. We need to honor truth, ours or another's, regardless if the expectations don't line up. When fear fuels a lack consciousness, we compromise ourselves and, as well, those we choose not deserving of our truth. I find selective truth one of the most insidious cop-outs around. It allows the perpetrator the ability to uphold an image of how they want to be represented in a given instance, portraying something different than the facts to another, because they feel unacceptable in their own heart. But like an addict, the fix in the moment overrides truth, and the façade is upheld. Disrespect, nonacceptance and dislike for self perpetuate.

In taking the path of least resistance by not speaking my truth, it may appear easier to keep things amiable, comfortable and seamless to avoid confrontation. In the interim it may provide respite, but speaks to a lack of trust in the potent, universal energy of cause and effect. It isn't the real deal, so begets more low vibrational outcomes. In practicing trusting in truth, I'm less capable to function in lazier ways of accepting what doesn't resonate within.

Shouldn't I at least attempt claiming the totality of my story, intending a clean and free will for self and others? Isn't acceptance for *what is* the very least we ask of each other, even if our perspective doesn't line up? So, why do we hesitate to lead as we would like to follow? Sure, it can initially feel solitary, standing solo as you start leading authentically, yet the alternative is following another instead of creating your own unique story. Then, you are not authentically giving to them, and so it goes. You cement your legacy each time you choose trusting in your own truth or not.

So, more questions as I move forward to whom I have in my life, why and what is driving it. What learning do I carry forward from perceived negative experiences? What negative energy needs untangling from combative situations? What resides beneath the anger? Lack of forgiveness is a good starter. Fear, envy and disappointment resist and dilute the power of a loving heart. What situations or individuals are not serving me and why do I carry them along? What does this say in terms of my sense of value and worth? What are the contrasts to these questions?

My ideal is to: evolve as a more loving, secure human being who compassionately engages in mutual truth; evolve, even if it requires taking responsibility for not doing right by another, even if without purposeful intention; evolve, mindful of consequences from my choices, now or later; and, evolve by not going to the dark, unhappy place to begin with.

Continue to build by living the questions. Build an abundant heart instead of creating a broken one, one truth at a time.

• • • • • • • • • • • •

> ♡ Being vulnerable doesn't have to be threatening. Just have the courage to be sincere, open and honest. This opens the door to deeper communication all around. It creates self-empowerment and the kind of connections with others we all want in life. Speaking from the heart frees us from the secrets that burden us. These secrets are what make us sick or fearful. Speaking truth helps you get clarity on your real heart directives.
> — Sara Paddison, *The Hidden Power of the Heart:*

Discovering an Unlimited Source of Intelligence

♡The ability to ask questions is the greatest resource in learning the truth.

— Unknown

. . . .

TAKE-AWAY PERSPECTIVE – DR. LEE PULOS

In a movingly open and transparent disclosure of her inner life while healing, Christine has demonstrated that as with drugs, success of surgery is partly dependant on our trust or "expectant faith." In study after study, patients with the most rapid healing following surgery – optimism and trust were the two most important attitudes to accelerate the healing response.

Sir William Osler, considered the greatest clinician and surgeon in the early 20th century, repeatedly stated that the cures he brought about were not due to any remedies applied but to the faith of the patients in treatment. Old ideas that germs and stress are the sole cause of illness have collapsed in the light of new evidence of how the intangibles of thoughts, beliefs and emotions have the greatest impact on health and well-being.

— Lee Pulos, Ph.D., ABPP
Clinical Psychologist
Author of *The Biology of Empowerment*
and *The Power of Visualization*
www.drpulos.com

vitalheart tip

Commit to living truthfully as your awareness and courage allow. The little lies and selective untruths create imbalance within. They reduce your sense of empowerment and true representation with others. You minimize connecting with like-minded, spirited individuals each time you choose a lie over the truth. The questions become:

- Why don't you value you enough to be truthful in this situation?

- What do you believe will change by being truthful?

- What is so threatening?

- How do you fully own your potential if unable to share the truth?

- How can another truly know and understand your essence if you do not bear your truth?

connect possibilities
body · mind · spirit · heart

INTERNET RESEARCH

International Society of Stress Studies....... www.istss.org

Self Empowerment Everyday Program ....
www.selfempowermenteveryday.com

Women's Health Every Day ..... www.everydayhealth.com

MUSIC

"A Day without Rain" .... www.enya.com

"December" .... www.georgewinston.com

"Stripped" .... www.christinaaguilera.com

READ

A Year by the Sea by Joan Anderson ... www.amazon.com

Self Matters by Dr. Phil McGraw........ www.amazon.com

The Heart's Code by Dr. Paul Pearsall ....
www.paulpearsall.com

Winds of Change by Stuart Wilde ... www.stuartwilde.com

HEAL

Calcium Magnesium liquid supplement . . . . Vitamin store

Traumeel - cream for scars. . . . . www.heel.com

Traumeel - electrolyte balancer . . . . www.heel.com

Vitamin shots . . . . Naturopath practitioner

chapter 4
fire in the belly

Adversity is simply a prelude to something more terrific to come. I grasp this notion for dear life hoping someday a fire in my belly will again ignite. It gives reason to attempt trusting in the wonders that life bestows upon us. It speaks to faith in truth and love, how they can and do conquer all that appears not so good with us.

So, I rewind to life pre-crumble . . . evaluating when, what and how I contributed in extinguishing my fire . . . leaving sparks and sputters with little oxygen to stoke a roar. My thought is by poking the embers where once a fire roared, perhaps it will spark new experiences. Then, a wide, sensational smile of *aha* will return to me, having acknowledged my learning.

In casting aside many warning signs of pre-crumble just three months ago, my ego *"push, make it happen, turn it around"* status quo maintained control from years of practice. In some respects it manifested incredible experiences, unique interactions and proud accomplishments. These adrenaline-fueled achievements perpetuated my overdrive mode whenever a so-called crisis or hurdle presented itself. Experience taught me I could figure *it* out with the right amount of "*go for it, Chrissie*" attitude.

However, the dark side of navigating in overdrive mode translated into a deceptive, slow depletion of stamina and, worse, unsound decision-making capabilities. My lack of sound judgment was certainly partially instrumental in *the crumble* circumstances. I compromised my truth by not trusting my worth, accepting an unhealthy threshold tolerance for pushing. This further weakened me by denial of the warning flags. How easily we delude and justify behaving in a manner that isn't our truth because we temporarily lack courage to value self. Eventually, this loops full circle, haunting us in one form or another.

One huge flag I chose to ignore was a particular episode on a late summer morning two months pre-surgery. I returned home exhausted and at odds of what to do after my weekly circuit exercise class. So, I climbed the stairs for a bath, which is my way to regroup. As I climbed, the energy literally flowed down and out my legs. Both limbs were drained of juice to move. With no choice but to succumb to the stairs, my head rested on one above while crouching on the one below until utter tiredness passed. It was a tiredness one can equate in having crossed the Ironman triathlon finish line—one not felt since, thankfully.

A withering vibrancy with internal and exterior signs flagged my need for shifts. An over-the-top superwoman façade for pumping out volumes of work each day was giving way to a cumulative exhaustion, which was present when I awoke and remained until sleep beckoned.

The more frequently I left the house sporting workout gear as the ensemble for the day, the more evident my lack of interest in appearance was due to overwhelm. During this period of time, even my designer jeans weren't getting equal wear time. With a reserve tank on empty, I justified the frenetic pace as doable given a healthy diet, lots of sleep, plenty of exercise and a nightly, healthy glass of vino. The internal mantra was, *"Just one more week, Chrissie, then you can restructure things, kick back and get rested up."*

Lack of laughter also signaled an imbalance. The odd spark of success was felt as periodic financial breathers occurred as sponsor monies were payable. I felt alone and very responsible to fulfill business obligations, to get solvent and develop a franchise-type model to sell—I saw this as a way out of the craziness I'd created. All this was in pursuit to work my life around career versus career around life, which was the norm to date. I cherished rare moments when harmony existed . . . sipping a mug of tea while delving into a novel that took me into another realm—cozy, safe, content.

* * * * * * * * *

"Freedom's just another word for nothing left to lose" sums up the post-crumble state of affairs toward the end of the year.

Cynicism by way of strong distrust and anger has replaced my immense passion and intellectual acumen formerly invested in my company. A few sparks barely keep everything lit. Ironically, the pacemaker regulates sparking my heart to beat regularly when the electrical system misfires . . .

Things are sputtering, at best. The question I constantly ask myself these days is, *"So, do you want to heal or not, Chris; that is, completely and on all levels?"* My struggle is to come to terms with the fact that despite best efforts and ridiculous amounts of *work* for a business, which truly ignited passion and purpose, the interim outcome is zip. Belief in the old adage of work really hard, do something you love, lead as you would like to follow and you will certainly enjoy the fruits of your labor is officially up for review. This premise almost killed me. I feel like a farce—the seminar series business owner who was preaching *owning your potential* barely makes it through her 42nd year.

Strong, motherly internal chats nudge me through this agonizing period of time, coming face to face with what I have or haven't created for my ideal. Inspired, happy thoughts are rare, though I'm grateful to be alive, most of the time. Being in a funk is bittersweet as it gives me the excuse to hang out and not push, which is good, yet I'm ever mindful of the potential for sliding into clinical depression. The loss of so much in a short period of time, plus dire financial circumstances can take anyone to their knees.

Anyone who says money isn't important has never looked up from the curb after investing heart, soul and financial credit into their passion. But, I keep punching as Dad always told us to do when the waters get rough. Or, perhaps, it's time to try another way by gently placing one foot in front of the other to test truth for *what is* . . . that I no longer can or want to push. I will trust being carried through.

I sputter along, taking each day in and of itself, just like an AA recruit. Physically, a rosy complexion returns to my cheeks, one absent since growing up. I wonder how long I battled with this condition. The doctors say it is congenital. So, an opportunity exists to let go and accept *what is*—way easier said than done, but necessary for my sanity.

Recovery workouts with the trainer are routine. My spirit resists any real enjoyment. I go through the motions knowing if I stop engaging in physical activity, fear will paralyze and I'll be hooped. I commit out of fear. One day, the trainer calls to cancel due to a flat tire; so, I commit to train solo, but nap instead— after a mug of tea and huge lemon tart. Anxiety wanes somewhat as stamina grows, but trepidation of arm movement prevails. I persevere with a bit of old push, which, in this scenario, works in my favor. Progress translates into sparks as one-hour non-stop workouts become easier. A core strength workout now takes a half versus one hour to complete. Stamina for the walk/run intervals reach 40 minutes, however, sadness and anger for having to build it up in the first place negates any sense of accomplishment.

Carson, my trainer, and I conquer a milestone with a seawall interval run/walk, but the experience is angst ridden. On the third interval, my legs and feet become jelly-like. I stop immediately. Carson encourages another four half-minute intervals, then a walk home up the hill. I feel drained on all fronts as we climb the hill while listening to his Pro Football career ending story—he can relate to my fear. His casual mention of counseling stays with me after I admit my emotionally fragile, defeated state.

Body weight is heading in a positive direction with a six pound gain to 135. I'm still underweight with a prior leanest being 140–145 given lots of muscle mass at 5'6". Weekly vitamin shots assist calming my nervous system, which results in a healthier weight. A new focus for cookbooks and fresh dishes occupies some time. I send Carson home with weekly meals as a thank you. He loves the home-cooked delicious experiments, made with pure heart.

⋆ ⋆ ⋆ ⋆ ⋆ ⋆ ⋆ ⋆ ⋆ ⋆

NOVEMBER – STRESS TEST

My scheduled stress test appointment arrives. The pacemaker nurse clarifies my condition is A/V Block, intermittent and idiopathic, meaning no known reason for it happening. The stress test appointment should be a snap.

Trauma gets hardwired quickly on a cellular level in one's body and can be triggered anytime without notice.

My day begins with mild anxiety—3 p.m. can't arrive soon enough. I enter the cardiologist's office with Carol. Compassion and grace are essential in this human interaction; however, I'm about to experience the polarized extreme. I need the comfort of another with me, partially because I feel so vulnerable and partially because the associated anxiety prevents me from absorbing everything said.

Thirty minutes in the waiting room and my a name is called. The nurse sets the tone with a curt *"no"* when I say Carol is joining me in the testing room.

"No, we don't want you in here in case something goes wrong," the nurse states and adds, "It's only because family usually cry or scream when something happens."

"Suck it up and dig deep, Chris; you will do this and be more than good to go," I recite to myself as internal panic wells up with an exterior calm.

The crazy thing about trauma is you don't know to what degree you've been traumatized until triggered at a later date. Waves of fear and emotion possess me as the two nurses converge on me. I suppose one might defend their lack of bedside compassion based on the repetition of this process, day after day. What a ridiculous notion to be mindful of *why* the patient is taking the stress test to begin with . . . not!

So, with trauma triggered, full-blown panic mode sets in; the frenetic-paced nurses hover like bees around the hive, attaching all sorts of electrical wires, sticky round pads and some waist belt, which is way too big, so keeps falling to the floor. My attempt to help is met with brushing my hand away without a word spoken; the blood pressure bands are next, which also fall to the ground—why can't they slow down to gently wrap things to fit? The only verbal dialogue I receive is when one sergeant major nurse, a wannabe jewelry maker, inquires who made my bracelet—I smirk a smidge of satisfaction that she isn't learned enough in her own craft to recognize a Tiffany's bracelet when she sees one.

They continue to buzz and move various limbs without a morsel of compassion. Angry and fearful, I think, *"Okay, make up your damn minds whether you want me to stand still or participate."*

Then, I am told, "I will conduct the test while she does some research, then, after that, you're going to be tested with another nurse who is also here today doing research."

I'm too maxed out to question when I agreed to be a research guinea pig as well as a pacemaker recipient. *"You can get through this, Chrissie, just focus on good things."*

I need to take responsibility for my welfare, so, with a tiny, shaky voice I share my nervousness for not having been on a treadmill since pre-surgery. I go on to share that the first time I knew something was amiss was almost passing out on the treadmill a few weeks ago. If they only knew what an admission of vulnerability this is for me. Neither throws me a bone, never mind an acknowledgement that I spoke.

I just need a soft human touch, a sense of being heard, and an acknowledgement that I'm in the room, not a number, but a human being in dire need of a spec of communal love. I feel so utterly alone in this experience, more so than the ER surgery day. I think but don't verbalize, *"You insensitive, cold bitches. I'd like to see how you'd handle this if the situation was reversed."* I reassure myself that anger is good, a vibrational step up from complete emotional collapse.

"Oh, you are in amazing shape and could probably stay on this thing for three hours," the sergeant major states from the laptop station. So, someone did hear me!

Again, I attempt to convey my need for reassurance. "Yes, well, my workouts since surgery are a max of 35 minute walk/runs with my trainer, just this last week."

Words fall on deaf ears with no response as one plays with a laptop. The familiar, uncomfortable beep, beep, beep signals the EKG monitoring humming into action.

I prod further for any information as my clammy palms tightly hold the treadmill sides.

"So, how long am I on the treadmill for? Will I be running or just walking?"

Another curt response, "As long as it takes you to MAX out."

"So what do you mean by maxing out?" Tears now trickle down my face.

"Oh, don't worry, we increase the speed every three minutes, and when you feel discomfort, you let me know."

I can't take anymore discomfort. I focus on my breath, trying to surrender to the fact I'm clearly on my own and can do this. I need to be brave for me.

"Okay, we're starting the treadmill," Nurse Ratchet spews.

My heart pounds. My internal buddy reassures me of the amazing runner I am. I try blocking out the cold, clinical disposition of the two *professionals*. Silent tears flow uncontrollably as the circumstances of the last six weeks and all that's transpired bubble to the surface.

At some point in stage three when the speed increases, a shortness of breath has me hopping to the treadmill side. It feels like trapped air, not out of breath from being winded. My breath returns to normal as soon as I jump off with no dizziness or other symptoms that would flag a problem. It all feels too much like the ER and I sob into my first post-surgery meltdown.

"Great, here sit down." Removal of the wires begins with no acknowledgement of my heaving sobs.

Finally, "Would you like a glass of water?" Another time, it would be humorous, so devoid of human compassion. I nod.

The other nurse finally connects with my eyes. "Don't you feel well, Christine?"

With an edge of cynicism and bewilderment of her cluelessness, I muster up, "No, I am fine. I am just very scared."

The nurse then hugs me saying, "It must have been quite a scare having this pacemaker put in."

I'm repelled by her display of compassion, seething with thoughts of *"too little, too late bitch—compassion, that is."* With nothing to give, I ponder what a shame as this experience had the potential to be inspirational and healing, if only I'd been treated as a human being instead of a rushed, late afternoon appointment.

The rest of the appointment is blurry as I go down the hall to my usual pacemaker nurse for regular tests and introductions to the pacemaker company representative. Her tender demeanor partially calms my shaking body as I continue to sob. My pal Carol holds my hand and mouths to me, *"Visualize good things."*

My voice is jagged and faint, "Maybe I'll come back another day when I'm calmer, to finish."

"We're almost done, so hang in there. This is a big milestone for you," she responds.

I focus on breathing through the rolling waves of panic while my legs shake uncontrollably.

Her parting words include: the stress test went well; the test's terrific; and, there's definitely a bereavement and grieving process with an experience of this magnitude. I thank her as I rush to leave, handing Carol my car keys—conceding to vulnerability.

Once home, though still shaking, the waves of panic slowly dissipate with a warm bath, a mug of tea, book in hand, and a cozy dinner with roommates and friends. I force my concentration to recall the many great memories in my life to date while a heart wrenching rawness, a deep sadness fills my being.

Things won't always unfold the way you want. Our choice is to react or respond, resist or let go. Individuals won't always "show up" the way you deem appropriate. Take time to get outside yourself whenever possible with compassionate words in approaching others. You never know what they're struggling with. Concentrate on keeping your heart open, period. Don't let others' tainted energy splash you.

Your moments of terror are incredible gifts if you can be brave enough to feel all you need to in the moment, regardless of how frightening and uncomfortable. It trumps the power of terror every time. This too shall pass. If you never have "dark" days, you'll never fully grasp effortless, magical days, which inspire and nurture the spirit.

This unfortunate experience has taught me the value in compassion. It softened some hard edges erected along the way. In witnessing the nurses' very unattractive, hard edges, my truth is to make a concerted effort to soften mine, so others don't bare the brunt of my misplaced anger and resentment. I believe this is what ages us from the inside out.

> ♡ In its infinite wisdom, the body remembers what the mind wants to forget, either consciously or subconsciously. It serves us symptoms that are important messages from our inner self about ourselves, what we are living out from the past and what changes in our life need to be made now if we are to heal and be healthy.
> — Niravi Payne, from *The Heart of the Healer*

. . . .

As I take inventory of my emotional, physical, financial and spiritual balance, apparently, a need to jump-start some sparks before all embers go out is upon me.

Emotionally, I consciously keep glumness at bay, so I don't slip into a depression not experienced so far in my life. Negative thoughts and words are frequent internal visitors and flag the need to energetically shift up, even if only from anger to frustration. My daily non-negotiable toward the positive spectrum is a bath, perfumed body lotion, and dressed in clean, fresh clothes by 10. I feel trickles of what dark depression is, and focus every bit of my energy on transforming it. It scares me to feel this low and sad. I have a new compassion for those who suffer from mental disorders.

Forced daily rituals help to up the ante. Daily journaling begins to rid my mountain of madness, triggering splinters of forgiveness for self and others. Internal coaxing away from high alert triggers slowly dampens my fire of irrational fear. A new book on dream analysis humors me as I awake from crazy, vivid dreams more often than not. The book states, *"If angels enter your home, you will be wealthy,"* so I hug this one close. The realization of my warped expectations of self and others reinforces the need to dissect all truths, small and large.

Redefining how I measure daily success results in a full breath when I permit the notion of not reaching for the stars every day. Practicing cruise mode when thinking I *should* be further along in healing is harder than it seems as I work to release self-judgment that others think I *should* be back on track. Internet research of heart-related conditions becomes a fascination and my fear wanes in tiny bits with new knowledge.

Financially, I come to terms with *what is*. Though not elated, at least I'm ready to deal in reality. A dear friend sums up my last years, "*You needed a wife.*"

I commit to work with a business coach to sort out the business finances while mapping out what's next for me. As well, I meet with a counselor whose response to current events is, "I would imagine you are reeling from it all."

Several conference calls with sponsors breathes peace when they're reassured I'm on the mend. Multiple lengthy conversations with my new business partner to map out the future provide me space to truly make the best decision for me. In admitting I no longer have any interest to raise operating capital, a burden is lifted for a truth silenced for a long while in the pursuit to keep the machine greased. This establishes the need to focus on gaining personal safety and predictability with a new income source.

Spiritual bankruptcy is proving harder to bounce back from than could've been imagined. In order to mend this malnourished soul, I try shifting perspectives a bit at a time. One journal entry attempts quenching my thirst to appease sorrow, *"I ask the divine to fill my body and spirit with the healing power of love strong enough that I can feel its power. I need this power so that I may heal and live my life fully in an anxiety-free manner."*

. . . .

The November chilly winter rain arrives and I welcome business coach Jeffrey Kearney's expertise. Our primary objective is to determine the future of the business and associated financial predicament. Once this game plan is handled, we assume some sense of order and safety will return so new possibilities can open up. Jeffrey's influence extends far beyond business negotiations to a complete evaluation of my values stemming from conscious and unconscious beliefs. This is the foundational framework for a refreshed ideal.

Tiny sparks sputter from the twisted chaos as one foot is placed in front of the other. The former mentality of go big or go home gradually gets reconsidered as my acceptance for *what is* surfaces an appreciation for simple basics—delicious food, plenty of sleep, inspiring conversation, reading to nurture the spirit, walks for tea to the café and the desire to relish in daily joys.

Sacred are our weekly one-hour coaching sessions. Within this space, I dabble in vitality, energy, truth and possibilities while letting my guard down to share the grief. His influence readjusts my fear-based perceptions including the possibility that running may be a worn-out activity with new ones to come. I reluctantly agree to consider this notion.

The premise of Jeffrey's work is to challenge one's current perspective, and, in turn, alter associated behaviors, actions and intentions, which no longer serve individuals or corporate cultures. His analogy is that, periodically, wet wood gets hauled around in the form of pre-existing beliefs, established systems, habits or attitudes that hold us back. Equally damaging is pushing a scenario along before its natural evolution by throwing a giant log on the fire when the kindling isn't even crackling. This results in a pitiful fire requiring little to blow itself out with absolutely no staying power. I've been famous for making things happen, an exhaustive endeavor. As well, it was arrogant believing I was so in control, having the wherewithal to actually make it happen. My resolve is to let go and let it be as is, which is taking plenty of awareness and practice in trusting this new way for being. Though very uncomfortable, this is my iron-clad commitment.

Jeffrey's aim in coaching is to "start the fire." So, how does he spark the kindling into a roaring blaze or ignite a spark that is barely lit? And, how does this truly, positively influence an individual or group?

He comments, "My job is to help a person or team find a perspective that gets the right kindling in place and ignites the fire at the right pace. Starting a fire . . . is first about igniting the spark. I love helping people and teams create that spark and tend it just enough so that it becomes self-sustaining. Lighting a fire is a threshold crossed. The spark represents the potential lingering below the surface of awareness."

Once sparked, this fire gets intense and causes significant, permanent change in individuals. Now, the individual(s) is accountable to engage individually and/or collectively to explore and evolve newly recognized potential for how it (the fire) can transcend their lives. He says, "I can't make people be any way. They have to choose who and how they want to be."

The following are some of the key insights I take away from my blessed time with him. They have influenced re-igniting my own fire within.

"Fear is both a motivator and a paralyzer. Paralysis is inaction. If I do nothing, stuff happens to me without my input or choice. If my choice is to work around it rather than work through it, then I stay stuck in fear, wondering if my work will really land or hold. When I become accountable for my fear and figure out a strategy on how to really address and deal with it, I get the inspiration and motivation I need to get moving."

How does one know when in the presence of someone nurturing their potential?

Jeffrey says, "They are not out to prove anything about themselves to others. They possess a sense of being grounded, an interest in others' input without desire for approval from them. Their passion tends to be internally driven. Their passion originates from what they are doing versus money being made. People in the artistic realm are examples of nurturing potential first for the love of it, creating something that inspires and is shared. An internal love for "it" resides. The money, recognition, etc., doesn't drive the effort, though it can be an amazing secondary benefit."

Jeffrey has become one of my favorite individuals to chat with, playing a priceless role in my life. His acumen has been instrumental in my systematically rebuilding various life aspects fueled from energetic passion instead of terror. Bit by bit, sparks ignite in my belly amidst great uncertainty.

I'm now tuned in to the difference in energy when sparks of truth and trust exists in conversations; this is when time flies by. It feels like a complete experience, which often resonates past the hour and the day, if super ignited. The beauty in this exchange lies in accessing potential for and with each other by sharing beliefs, experiences and feelings. It is enthusiastic, authentic, intentional and attentive because both parties are present.

My current truth is that I need to cultivate a new, softer way of being in this world. The strong ego push is worn-out and needs balancing out to appease struggle. The truth is I disassociated from the surgery and other contributors to *the crumble* to avoid this present pain. The stress test snapped me out of denial and into a sewer of raw emotions. It looks like there is trauma to heal.

A book I recently read states that trauma results in heightened sensory and perceptual emotions. So, I guess the dizziness and light-headedness experienced when repeatedly relaying *the crumble* story signals that my detachment to the pain is wearing thin. My business partner's astute observation of my present circumstances are bang on "you are not living your values" and "your past pattern is making decisions that don't align with your values, in that you can't fulfill them and that creates strife."

If not now, then when will I spark another fire in my belly?

When was the last time you felt the ignited spark? Next time you speak your truth, see what ignites to move you forward. Trust the spark and nurture it with honor and respect.

> ♡ Do the thing you fear to do and keep on doing it . . . that is the quickest and surest way ever yet discovered to conquer fear.
>
> — Dale Carnegie

TAKE-AWAY PERSPECTIVE – MIRABEL PALMER ELLIOTT

Christine starts this chapter with "Adversity is simply a prelude to something more ideal to come." That echoes my experience too. I've been through enough adversity by now to know that it is always an access to seeing something new and powerful.

Twenty years ago, I was severely injured in a car accident. I had just been married, and was on a fast-paced career path to success. Suddenly my world devolved into chronic pain and nothing but physio and rehab. After months of this, and hints that I was heading into depression, my doctor handed me a research study saying that 97 percent of people who miss more than six months of work due to an accident never return to full-time work or rigorous physical activity again. Even amidst depression and months of chronic pain, I was clear I was not interested in that prognosis. I created a new career that allowed me to return to work at a pace I dictated. I recently completed a ten-year stint working very full time as a senior director with Rogers. I also began a very simple exercise regimen to get myself physically back on my feet. I now work out six days a week, ski like a maniac, including competing in moguls, and, at 48, I'm in the best physical condition of my life.

About five years ago, I took a personal development course that altered my life in ways I'd never imagined possible. I learned in this course, the Landmark Forum, that in any place in our life where we experience struggle, there is something we are not telling the truth to ourselves about (or as Christine has pointed out, we are not acting consistent with our truth). Once we get clear about that and take responsibility for what we've been telling ourselves, there is access to a new perspective we couldn't see before. And that leads to new possibilities opening before us, or, as Christine's would say, to new potential. Through the Landmark Forum I've had access to new possibilities in areas all over my life—areas where I've lacked power for years, and areas that were already going well; my career, my relationship with parents, husband and kids, and many others.

What I now see is that after my car accident, I was operating inside the perspective that I'd lost everything. In fact, when I look back even before the accident, to the days of my stellar career, underneath the success was a constant battle with this belief that I was a loser. Once I saw that, I had a choice to create a new perspective. I chose a perspective of possibility. Suddenly a once bleak future had openings in it. Do I still experience that old nagging thought that I'm a loser every once in a while? You bet. And every time it crops up, it's an access to new possibilities—something more ideal to come.

— Mirabel Palmer-Elliott
Partner and Social Architect
Social Energy www.socialenergy.ca
e-mail: Mirabel@socialenergy.ca

vitalheart tip The next time you feel particularly challenged, take a few minutes out, grab a tea and reflect on the worst day you ever endured, and the best day you've experienced to date. What gifts were bestowed to you from the worst day? Now, take those gifts, recollect the feelings of the best day and carry all of it with you for the rest of today.

connect possibilities
body · mind · spirit · heart

INTERNET RESEARCH

Heart Math Institute . . . . www.heartmath.org

Findhorn Foundation . . . . www.findhorn.org

Mayo Clinic Newsletter . . . . www.mayoclinic.com

Nightingale-Conant . . . . www.nightingale.com

Real Age Newsletter . . . . www.realage.com

READ

A Dog's Life by Peter Mayle . . . . www.amazon.com

Feel the Fear and Do it Anyway by Susan Jeffers . . . .
www.amazon.com

Leadership from the Inside Out by Kevin Cashman . . . .
www.amazon.com

Transitions by William Bridges . . . . www.amazon.com

chapter 5
yin & yang, the balancing act

Yin and Yang energy is the duality of the same whole, the do and be energies. Yin is the feminine energy characterized by trust, flow, love, connection, intuition, inner wisdom, birth, softness, truth. On the other hand, Yang energy is characterized by getting things done, the pragmatic mind, aggressive, focused, physical strength and task oriented. The ideal is for human beings to blend the two energies to create harmony, internally and externally. My hair grows out with soft curls framing a renewed Yin side.

Spring has arrived in true West Coast fashion with a rainy, cold drizzle. It's Vancouver after all. Six months post-surgery and my mood of late matches the wet, gray cold weather outside. There exists an apathy and restlessness, which makes me feel a tad loopy. I am stuck.

Fun and ease don't depict the past six months. I know I'm accountable for what is or is not showing up in my world no matter how tough my recent challenges were. There's a need to learn an easier way to navigate. I now get that my unhealthy push, which defined me until *the crumble*, represented an imbalance of Yin and Yang energy. My Yang (masculine) energy dominated with fierce independence and a *can do* mantra. My newly acquired vulnerability shows me a healthier way to accomplish with ease of heart and spirit, the Yin energy. The truth is I need to cultivate the Yin to soften my edges and create an ease craved over a lifetime.

My body lets me know when moving with Yin energy as a feeling of balanced ease and quiet power guides me with a lighter step. I certainly want to cherish my Yang acumen and negotiation skills to ensure things get handled. My learning is to dance with both energies equally.

> ♡ Learning how to access a continuity of common sense can be one of your most efficient accomplishments in this decade. Can you imagine "common sense" surpassing science and technology in the quest to unravel the human stress mess? In time, society will have a new measure for confirming truth. It's inside the people—not at the mercy of current scientific methodology. Let scientists facilitate discovery, but not invent your inner truth.
> — Doc Childre, *Self-Empowerment: The Heart Approach to Stress Management*

For me, *to-do lists* spell security and comfort when perceiving a lack of order, uncertainty. They're my way of making sense of things, motivating myself beyond procrastination when stuck, to witness tangible progression in striking it *off the list*. If you've never tried the list thing, you should at least once. The instant gratification in striking an item off the list is terrific. My list-making technique started when I coproduced an international sports event for 80,000 spectators years ago. The details within each area of my overall responsibility became overwhelming with nightly "event mares" waking me. I tamed this internal chaos through lists, removing the chaos within my head to minimize the incessant worry and dwelling. I wish I'd pioneered the 3M stickem as they are the best on-the-go mini list ever created. Lists are certainly Yang based.

Those near and dear often tease me for my mundane errands list, but it helps keep my head clear and we are rarely out of milk, toothpaste or wine. It's just more effortless to jot it down and let it go until in the car and on my way.

I've lived list free for the better part of the past six months, nurturing a Yin way. However, balance is essential, so I reinstate lists on a trial basis as renewed interest in stepping out emerges. Apathy and restlessness prompt this call to action and my hope is to take the good parts of my Yang forward as my Yin begins to balance it with grace. I miss a creative outlet and associated electric brainstorm sessions, which inspired many business visions. I miss the thrill of chaos resolved when a collective mastermind group creates better options through intellect, experience and intuition. I miss the sense of reward in sourcing and receiving new funds of $100,000 plus made out to my business name. And, I have absolutely zero interest in stirring the chaotic push pot again, to the best of my conscious awareness.

So, I set out to create a Yin-Yang list to stimulate my feminine and masculine attributes with new truths. I want to be able to say I'm active, fully functioning, and balanced with minimal residual trauma and fear tainting the possibilities.

The Yin and Yang lists evolve on new terms.

1. Yin – Research writing information and classes to write a book

2. Yin – Sign up for belly dancing (this will be fun and sensual)

3. Yin – Commit to exploring Buddhist lectures and meditation at the library

4. Yang – Free myself from the fear of working out and not running

5. Yang – Resolve financial predicament with business and start earning

6. Yin and Yang – Clean bill of health for six-month cardiology checkup

7. Yin – Define the ideal for relationships and seek a mentoring role

8. Yang – Grow *Own Your Potential* business concept to develop a column

9. Yin – Love is in the Air

LIST ITEM #1

Contacting the local author's group isn't effortless or energizing, so I course correct, and resource library books to play with book outlines for some brewing concepts. This is a terrific admission of truth for my love of the written word as a reader and budding writer. I simply love the smell of books, certain types of paper, the font, the clever covers, and the way great stories propel my growth, introducing new perspectives.

This task triggers a new fear in not trusting *me* to uphold the pact to maintain balance. My past experience has been an all-or-nothing approach when passion of any kind comes knocking, thereby, ultimately costing me. I don't know how to create business projects without them taking over, so I start to trust *listening* when to step sideways. And, tap, tap, tap away, I write conceptual outlines despite resistant fear. Fear is so irrational for the most part, so you need to let it know you hear it and then gently tell it to buzz off.

· · · · · · · · · · ·

LIST ITEM #2

I always saw belly dancing as a highly feminine, sensual way to move one's body. In an effort to dust mine off, that is sensuality, I commit to this physical activity. I hope it will help conquer my air bubbles (fear) with pure fun to fully land in my body. It proves to be an absolute hoot. What I witness is the larger, more full-bodied women in the class are more at ease with sensual ways than some of us lean, athletic lot. Being athletic, my moves are initially awkward, but give way to sourcing a softer, more feminine aspect, which I love. My pal, Cathy, joins me for the weekly class and it soon becomes a weekly evening out with vino after at a local restaurant bar. The bar regulars get apprised of our latest moves and the hysterical play by play of our recital debut to a clapping crowd of 200 plus. Terrific new memories and the most fun in ages are had. I love Cathy's *go for it* attitude with oodles of belly laughs to boot.

· · · · · · · · · · ·

LIST ITEM #3

I bite the bullet and attend a community library Buddhist lecture. Christine, the teacher, leads us with a mix of meditation, group discussion and teachings. She is gentle, animated and humorous in her delivery. I want to emulate her demeanor in all I do. I *know* this is a solid decision. I grow to crave the weekly nurturing hits of calm and insights, no matter how tentative I feel that day.

I notice subtle shifts I like and am proud of the peace and humility cultivated each week. More often than not, I arrive in a civilized pace with time to spare. My past schedule was accounted for to the minute, which left me wired and unable to fully take a breath. I notice moments of restlessness are about stirring things up when a surplus of peace and ease exist. This insight is revealed in the quiet. Instant panic ensues when I feel periodic chest healing pains where my muscle was cut, so I learn to sit in the pain and breath, trusting that *this too shall pass*. This muscle pain takes two years plus to heal, so each time it surfaces, I practice in-the-moment breath. A slight shift happens whenever I'm aware of negative chatter and choose to replace delusions with positive thoughts. I notice random thoughts about creating a new column. It feels doable and I don't sense pressure but a healthy challenge and, dare say, a bit of excitement.

Not every meditation class experience is peaceful. Three weeks into going for Buddhist hits, I plunk down in *my* spot at the back of the room with my back to the wall. Rushes of extreme raw emotions come out of nowhere. I had deliberated coming, but knew if I just got here, peace of mind and ease would reward me. Puddles of tears gush while another Buddha enthusiast extends me the sweetest gesture, handing me tea before pouring his own. With this gesture, I feel the transformative heart of human kindness in being watched out for. My puddles eventually dry out and I connect with a collective belonging within the four walls of this class. The truth is I want to manifest this collective belonging as a core value in all parts of my life. I can create it by first giving it—love.

One question posed in group discussion is, "How do you know when the mind has truly let go of 'it,' the emotion attached to the delusion of mine or another?"

The teacher's response, "You have a feeling of lightness and peace, not neutral as that indicates no action or feeling, but peace and lightness, an internal smile."

So, I try lightness in heart and spirit to absolve the powerful demons, one by one. Edginess lingers within spirit for a long time post-crumble, but without fail, my mood is transformed upon saying good-bye to my fellow Buddhas in training as I depart from my sacred time at the library. For months, it is the one time I open the car moon roof to blast out music and sing my way home while tears of hopeful viability spill. These brief glimpses in feeling quiet excitement and happiness let me know that anything is still possible. The weekly hits feed my soul.

* * * * * * * * * *

LIST ITEM #4

Feel the fear and do it anyway, Chrissie! I haven't set foot in the training gym yet and, given that past running buddies are nowhere to be seen, I decide to venture back on a particularly dreary rainy day. At 3:30 p.m., I'm dressed, apprehensive and determined. Oodles of demons swirl away after not being able to reach even one friend to say, *"You know, today I am not as brave as other days. Will you join me for a half hour at the gym for a walk/bike?"* I am discouraged and feel like a wimp for needing support.

4:40 p.m. rolls around. After numerous lame excuses, I've now circled the gym block three times. Finally parked, I breathe in the familiar waft of gym air while being welcomed by the trainers with open arms. Fresh tears of surrender, joy and praise spill on the dried sweat beads of the gym floor. I admit to the trainers feeling shear terror as I plug in earphones blasting SEAL. I hop on the treadmill for the first time since the stress test. I internally negotiate and commit to 25 minutes of walk/run intervals at level 3.0, which gets bumped up to 3.3 the last five minutes. A tight thud in my upper torso washes over me at minute 23 as I break a sweat, so I slow down and walk the remainder. It feels like trapped air.

"Each time it will get easier, right now, it's only about feeling good," I coach myself.

This is a huge victory and, now, a Tuesday afternoon routine begins at the gym. Soon after, I take in a weekend yoga class to nurture new acquaintances and appreciation for this sort of physical, soulful activity.

Around this period of time, I welcome the most unlikely of running buddies into the mix. Mary and I ponder the possibility of doing a 5k run on my one-year surgery anniversary. We begin weekly walk/run times at the soccer field and eventually progress to the seawall.

The weekly recovery workouts are elevated with boxing gloves. My trainer, Carson, arrives with boxing gloves knowing I previously loved boxing at the gym. Trepidation seizes my body, my neck and shoulders tighten like a vice. I override the fear to get over myself and go for it. My right arm definitely gives the better punch! Then, in a flash, I stop and blurt out in a panicked voice that the nurse said no to boxing. Carson talks me off the ledge, reassuring me that the leads attached to my pacemaker won't spring from my chest. The nurse was referring to contact boxing and getting hit in the chest. This makes sense, so I breathe, relax and refocus to draw strength from each punch. It spurs me forward, though I'm a bit rattled by the terror that erupted from deep within without warning. Carson leaves with his weekly meals-to-go. I prepare them with respect, love and gratefulness for his presence in my world.

LIST ITEM #5

The "banksters" get reconciled. A pal of mine, Margaret owns a company that helps others sort through their debt problems, offering various resolves. She has guided me along as to my options given the current financial crisis. I decide to close my business, which interestingly isn't too emotional. I know it's a detour and something will seed from this debacle of sorts. My only hesitation is the lost opportunity to work with my business partner. He truly is integrity, heart in action and wickedly smart. My loss, but, hopefully, one day he will read this and know I'm wiser and very grateful for his brief but influential role in my life. As well, I surrender because the associated financial fallout is about to take me out unless I shift perspective to keep juggling all to work.

Gaining a positive perspective proves easier said than done. I'm disillusioned in having leveraged all personal credit in anticipation of long-term financial equity from five years of sweat equity. It is obvious that without investor funding, the business can't grow. I lack the courage, or, perhaps, am wiser about financially extending myself or, more importantly, my new business partner. I cannot consciously put Don in a position of financial risk given my fragile and compromised mindset. I don't trust my ability business wise right now. This is a first and I feel extremely dependant and needy all of a sudden. I need to stop the bleeding so it won't drag anyone down.

My options are to go bankrupt or try to negotiate a deal with trustees. I chose the trustee route as it allows me to earn and keep any income level. Bankruptcy takes everything after the first $1,500 net per month and, therefore, leaves one paralyzed and morally in a state of poverty. In addition to my recent challenges, of equal importance is the lack of empowerment I know I'll feel with bankruptcy. So be it then if a walloping monthly payment is the cost to regain empowerment and ensure freedom of income—the lesser of two evils. I'm making decisions and believe they are in everyone's best interest. It's a point of distinction and integrity.

Negotiating with the banksters since *the crumble* for outstanding lines of credit and credit card balances reinforces how fragile I feel. This unnerves me and is excruciatingly uncomfortable, yet I can't shake free of it. My business negotiating skills are still intact, but absorb what little reserve energy is left. I learn to pick my battles wisely. When collection agencies call, I hang up as I can't afford any negative interactive dialogue.

A trustee works on my behalf . . . or is it the creditor's behalf? This is a conundrum not yet resolved with me. A proposal is put forth to all creditors for around 20 cents on the dollar. The day of reckoning arrives and the largest creditor, the tax man, is present for the meeting. The mere thought of entering a corporate office, never mind negotiating my cause, gives me reason to crawl under a duvet to be eternally comforted. I call on Dad to come with me, no longer attempting any *make it happen* ability. I need moral support, which is bittersweet as it makes me feel more screwed up having asked. In hindsight, I realize the dance with Yin and Yang is perfected on this day. I'm learning to trust in the power of the feminine Yin energy. The truth is I don't want to do life on my own anymore.

Dad sips several coffees in a street café while I plead my case 15 floors up at the trustee's office. The Coles/CliffsNotes version is: I agree to pay $800 monthly for more years than is tolerable. In return, I don't go bankrupt, so I can earn any income amount. My *make it happen* trait works in my favor today. It will make cameo appearances as the situation warrants over time. I earned this Yang energy through pure grit from years in business and am proud of this acumen.

The *suits* outline the terms and then, in a very out of character gesture, inquire what my new gadget means for my future. Initially I am shocked by the humane gesture. Intuitively I stumble into what feels appropriate to share—my truth. I reveal amazing technology facts, the short surgery time and the ability to run tomorrow if I want. Then, for some reason, I offer to show my pacemaker. All are super keen and intrigued. A very human and humbling interaction equalizes all. We all know where the real power truly resides within the room at this moment. Standing up at the boardroom table, I unbutton my blouse enough for the pacemaker peep show and encourage the *suits* to touch it. In leaving, my perspective has shifted to one of observing individuals just doing their job to collect a pay check. They, like you and I, are starved for truthful encounters void of forced policies and systems, which stifle uniqueness, productivity and profit. Their faces literally softened with compassion and interest in what truly mattered this day—individuals mutually caring for and respecting one another first and foremost.

With the peep show finito, Dad and I share in a hysterical laugh at the absurdity of it all while driving home. This is one for the books! The hysterical laugh was a façade for coming off of what would be the last time I'd set foot in a densely-aired, contained, toxic corporate environment. A spark of empowerment is ignited in having trust to speak my truth of vulnerability. I am much stronger than I think I am.

. . . .

LIST ITEM #6

My six-month pacemaker checkup appointment arrives. I feel as relaxed as I can expect. Jackie, the nurse, inquires how the workouts are going. She knows how vital this is to my emotional healing. I hear the catch of emotion in my voice. A raw sadness pervades for all I've dug out from under. I also understand more intimately what I am made up of with pride. We share laughs as I choke back tears. I feel robbed of assumed, youthful physical strength and love for athletic prowess, which is no longer psychologically effortless and enjoyable. And, so it is for today. With my friend, Carol, in tow, we celebrate six months of paced health with a lavish high tea at Urban Tea Merchant followed by shopping at Lululemon. I'm relieved not having to step back in this office for another year.

LIST ITEM #7

Relationships are defined for life-long propositions. A veneer of sadness comes over me when one of my longest, dearest friends crosses my mind, which is often. This kinship went by the wayside along with *the crumble*. With a protective armor enveloping my heart strings, I accept the 20-year friendship needs to naturally cease to exist if that is what is to be. I'm not angry per se, just resigned to seeing the truth as it is now. We experienced great highs and lows together, sometimes simultaneously. This is not the first time our friendship was tested when my chips were down. Clearly, my expectations are out of whack and I'm choked at the insensitivity of it all. And, it's all good. Presently, I'm not the strong one and accept not everyone is comfortable witnessing one they love in such a state. Vulnerability is so often mistaken for weakness, an invaluable insight gained from my own circumstances. I get it but it doesn't make it acceptable to me. She lent me money to help me through this rough patch and, one day, I will return it as promised. I'll always be grateful to her for this gift. I can love her from afar and wish her only the best. She was the one I believed I'd witness the end of this lifetime with.

I explore mentoring and adoption options. It's time to step outside myself to unconditionally serve another with much love. I wonder what this or, rather, who this will look like?

LIST ITEM #8

The abundance concept is simple, yet we complicate it so easily. My understanding is we need to practice the abundance mode all the time, particularly in moments when despair and scarcity seem copious. It's a no brainer to embrace the Law of Attraction premise when all is flowing, but we human beings seem to take leave of our senses when things are headed toward lack. So, I *work* to stay in the abundance mindset when served up what feels like a bowl of lack.

Ruthie, a heaping helping of feminine abundance, arrives at my door. I've grown to have immense regard for this woman's acumen and adore her understated femininity of spirit. We first met when she represented a company sponsoring my seminar series. She came across sharp as a tack with a get-down-to-it, East Coast business style. She mirrored my masculine energy and I wasn't entirely comfortable with it. Overtime, we revealed a more feminine side to one another and have become friends beyond the initial business acquaintance. I continue to be awed by who shows up for me, ones like Ruthie who I least expect to demonstrate their love in action, their version of authentic care.

"Observe the situation. Observe your response. Observe another's response. Observe your response."

In true Ruthie style, she arrives with champagne and suited in perfected East Coast chic attire—demure, elegant with a twist of hip sass. In observing what I say, do and don't do, she offers fabulous insights and wisdom to spur me onward. Her words insist creating my next bliss and begin today. She prods me to create something from the writing portion of my business. She teases me to permit getting jazzed up again, and stresses it doesn't need to be big. She questions if I trust in my value, saying, "Only then, will your confidence and trust return." Finally, she tells me to let go of unhealthy responsibility to all involved in the seminar series—that life happens and we all move on.

And so, the seed of my "Own Your Potential" column is germinated this night. It sparks a creative purpose once again! I realize in holding myself back to prevent my old push, I've created an apathetic mood. I need to trust keeping myself in check and gauge current truth on how I manage this. Ruthie ends up offering me a monthly column on a national health-oriented company website. And so, my writing muse begins in earnest ...

I've learned much from Ruth along the way and, though our contact is sporadic, I'm so fortunate for taking the time to really get to know the human being behind the corporate face. She is a blessing to me.

* * * * * * * * * * *

LIST ITEM #9

Love is in the air, spring that is. I slowly glue bits of my shattered heart together from the last romance. I take 100 percent responsibility as I chose to participate in a situation that wasn't in my highest good, so feel no malice or criticism toward my romantic interest. It is what it is—a painful lesson with shame still front and center, but perhaps a necessity to bring focus on what I truthfully want this part of my life to look like.

Until now, I enjoyed plenty of romance as an a la carte item to my career. Now, I want to create a lifestyle first, where family is primary with career built around it. The pacemaker awoke me to the fact I probably waited too long to have babies and, now for the first time, I feel the maternal clock ticking. My intuition tells me that physically it is probably best to leave well enough alone. Why did I wait so long? There were many opportunities. It's hard to fathom finishing this life without experiencing giving birth to my own child. I would be a really good mom. Tears silently spill when I see a newborn in a mother's embrace. I don't believe it's possible to emulate this type of connection in another way. The pain of not experiencing it tugs at my heartstrings. It is another reminder to start living truth for all that I want in life.

I see no harm in enjoying male company if a clear understanding of no physical intimacy is conveyed and mutually agreed upon. I want to attract a man to become an integral part of my life when I'm stronger, when I possess renewed confidence and positive momentum. I don't want to attract someone in my current state where vulnerability and neediness are the norm versus the exception. It's not the role I'm interested in playing with my equal.

I venture out socially a bit more for the odd glass of vino at the pub with friends and quasi dates here and there—all good individuals. I take time to truly determine what aspects I need and want in the next Mr. Right.

Spring showers come and go. With the showers is apathy to commit to either the darkness of winter or blooms of summer—the perfect analogy for my emotions. My resistance to the old masculine ego push has been trying, and my persistence to find a softer, more feminine way begins blossoming into an easier way, absent of unhealthy adrenaline.

John Maher has a great line in his song "Split Screen Silence" that speaks to what I would convey to Mr. Romance gone sideways if I saw him now, *"it's all right, you got your heart right."* It's not ready for intimacy yet, but my romantic heart is right now with lessons learned, splinters removed and healing with renewed love for self.

* * * * * * * * * *

TAKE-AWAY PERSPECTIVE – CHRISTINE BROWN

Without inner peace, outer peace is impossible.
For true lasting happiness, trust in truth!
Trust=Faith
Truth=Dharma (i.e., Buddha's teachings)
Trusting in truth= Faith in dharma!
Buddha's teachings
(Quotes extracted from *Transform Your Life* by Geshe Kelsang Gyatso)

Happiness and suffering are states of mind, and so their main causes cannot be found outside the mind. The real source of happiness is inner peace. If our mind is peaceful, we shall be happy all the time, regardless of external conditions, but if it is disturbed or troubled in any way, we shall never be happy, no matter how good our external conditions may be.

If we want true, lasting happiness, we need to develop and maintain a special experience of inner peace. The only way to do this is by training our mind through spiritual practice—gradually reducing and eliminating our negative, disturbed states of mind and replacing them with positive, peaceful states.

If we first establish peace within our minds by training in spiritual paths, outer peace will come naturally; but if we do not, world peace will never be achieved, no matter how many people campaign for it.

— Christine Brown, Meditation Teacher
Tilopa Buddhist Centre, BC, Canada
www.kadampa.org

vitalheart tip — Each night as you tuck into bed, take the first few moments to quietly breathe in gratefulness for all the wonders of your day, small or large. You will be surprised at how many things you are thankful for.

connect possibilities
body · mind · spirit · heart

INTERNET RESEARCH

Global Community Thinkers................www.ted.com

Kadampa Buddhism ....www.kadampa.org

International Women Writing Guild ....www.iwwg.com

READ

Wouldn't Take Nothing for My Journey Now
by Maya Angelou .... www.amazon.com

Why People Don't Heal and How They Can
by Caroline Myss .... www.amazon.com

LISTEN

"Lost my Belief" by SEAL (Music)............www.seal.com

DO

Belly Dancing.................... Local Community Center

Personal Trainer .... Local Fitness Facilities

chapter 6
owning your potential

Action mode is the name of the game as I reach the half-year mark from *the crumble*. Aspirations are surfacing, though the action part is far from effortless as I commit to engage, explore and evolve through this muck. Uncertainty spells fear for me, so I continue to practice surrender to *what is* from the crumble by trusting in a higher purpose for all that occurred.

If I just stay attuned for the lessons and retain what still works from the way I use to do and be, then my shattered heart bits will heal, on my own terms. There is no question I'm evolving into a more compassionate, grounded and secure individual since being stripped to the core of previous, material trappings. A core worth, based entirely on how much you attain or have amassed will drop you to your knees in a moment if your soul isn't sound in inherent value. So, I learn that I have a ways to go to value this soul. AND, I possess an inner strength and sense of self that will carry me through to lightness in due course.

The year progresses and I enjoy tangible evidence of many germinating ideals. With patience and trust, I reap a few harvests before year end: my column is launched; my one-year surgery anniversary is celebrated by participating in a 5k run/walk; my business head begins percolating other ways to innovate with like-minded connectors; my financial plan involves trading down my caliber of automobile, a temporary sidestep; my interim income projects include, amongst other projects, a paper route with Dad, the retired judge; my want to mentor in lieu of children is granted, I meet a girl who I nickname Pippi.

> The greatest truth must be recognition that in every man, in every child is the potential for greatness.
> — Robert Kennedy

. . . .

I launch the "*Own Your Potential*" column in the fall. The column vision is: a desire for readers to be responsible for their inherent intuition to elevate potential; a desire to take the best parts of my business forward to explore possibilities; a desire to profile the many experts I cultivated business relations with; and a desire to honor my quiet, strong voice that spoke *"write a book"* while I lay on the ER gurney. I *know* these columns are the precursor.

When writing the column, any incessant, negative internal chatter comes to a full halt. The truth is I love the written word. It feels like magic in this medium. Reader feedback of any sort is exhilarating as it proves my writing is manifesting dialogue with shared opinions. It doesn't even matter if it is confrontational. In fact, this is good, as it stretches my biased perspective. The feedback reinforces I've created a forum of engaged readers and, so, my purpose is fulfilled!

The column also gives me the excuse I feel is needed to reconnect with exceptional individuals from my business. It relieves an underlying sense of guilt in closing the business. John Stanton, owner of the international chain The Running Room, is one of these individuals. He is one of the first individuals interviewed for the column. "Unassuming" best describes him.

His sentiments on when his world crumbled are, "Crumbles are speed bumps in life and these *s*peed bumps provide the opportunity to learn about ourselves and individuals we've chosen to surround ourselves by." John refers to his pre-Running Room days as *"the guy who spent a lot of time on the couch after long days in a sales job—tired, out of shape and, mostly, not satisfied with his own potential."* Now, John is sporting loads of fun. "It is hard to distinguish between work and play and that's the way I like it."

Care and respect are two core values John embraces. He focuses on three wins; 1k, 5k, and 10k success markers. The 1k marker is about foundational life-long goals to work at something considered play. The 5k marker is about enjoying the people he works with and creating wins for them. The 10k marker is about building community with a coaching camaraderie through run and walk clinics hosted by his stores—he literally runs with this three-way win theory!

I receive his congratulations in signing up for a 5k run this fall. I was participating in his half marathon race group through one of his retail outlets when surgery interfered a week prior, so we both get what this run means for my psyche.

"Find the possibilities," is Mirabel Palmer-Elliott's mantra to evolve potential. Mirabel championed my business vision by negotiating

Chatelaine, a national magazine for the title sponsor role during the last few business years. It transformed my business, the seminar series into a national proposition. Our relationship grew from a surface business type to an entrusted friendship when we spoke our respective truth during one particular conference call, which was mutually exasperating.

We both trusted enough in the mutual end goal to navigate through the tenuous conversation to share our truth. We respected one another's acumen. It was a courageous, refreshing act of alliance in a corporate environment. This dynamo keeps evolving through whatever comes her way. Her most influential daily action is awareness to find possibilities in negative or challenging situations. She consciously invents the possibility by attention to and intention for how she desires the day to unfold.

Mirabel practices this process so it will become second nature. Her questions to another when pondering their potential are:

- What is the possibility for you to own more potential for a something or someone?

- Why are you not exploring it?

- If the attainment of this something or someone could translate into evolving more of your potential, then what are you waiting for?

- Are you fixated on a specific desired outcome or unsure if you can achieve it instead?

- Are you indulging in the mystery of possibilities by engaging in the process now?

* * * * * * * * * * *

Along came Mary. A chronic residual crumble fear is running. I literally think I'll keel over; perhaps die given the only warning flag of anything amiss was dizziness when working out. Mary, a long-time acquaintance is a pleasant surprise who checks in to see how I'm managing.

One particularly low day, I admit with extreme embarrassment of my fear in running. On the spot, Mary suggests twice weekly runs for a 5k race on my one-year surgery anniversary. Many 7 a.m. mornings, I'm too depressed to contemplate such an activity, but I haul my sorry, fearful and, now, giggly butt out of bed hoping courage will surface by the time I meet her at the seawall.

I used to run this seawall four times weekly without a care in the world. Courage doesn't always show up but Mary does. She inspires me to run through my fear with a gentle approach by coaxing me one runner in front of the other. She isn't a seasoned runner. She enlightens me through her actions in the power of compassion. She nudges me along many mornings when I am so miserable for not being able to run like pre-surgery days that I can barely stand running with me! I didn't know I could be so miserable.

We complete the race on October 1, one year to the day from last year's surgery. One of the trainers from the gym comes along to support us. Mary is ecstatic. I am surprised by my lack of any strong emotion. My expectations are obviously still out of whack. Later, I realize that I'm so busy being pissed in doing the walk/run intervals, instead of running like one short year ago for the race, that I miss the present gift in this milestone. After all, one year prior, I was lying in the ER fighting for my life and now I've just finished a 5k race, but there is no comforting me.

I let myself and Mary down on this day, though not intentionally. The disappointment and judgment in her eyes devastates me. I can't articulate what is going on within, but *it* won't permit me to celebrate this accomplishment. It's as though I won't feel accomplished until experiencing a pre-surgery type of run. We lose touch and stop running after this event . . . I am not upset with her—she just couldn't look beyond what her and my expectations were for me that day. Another lesson learned.

* * * * * * * * * * *

Relinquishing ego, practicing resiliency and getting resourceful come to mind about my paper route stint this fall. I experience a big ego hit with drastic lifestyle changes due to my current economic misfortune. This tests my trust in the Law of Attraction theory as belief in abundance is hard to envision, never mind touch right now. In order for this law to work its magic, I need to believe, to trust in my desire no matter what the circumstances are. My financial circumstances are dire. I feel enormous burden and responsibility to shift this brutal way of seeing everything through a dark cloud each day. But, the reality is: my $800 monthly payment to the trustee is $800 more than is coming in; my beloved Audi has to get traded down for a Jetta; my weekly splurge is limited to a measly glass of wine out and, twice weekly, Chai Lattés after walks at the beach with Rudi; my ability to get a corporate gig is psychologically out of the question, so I need to resource a unique solution.

On top of this financial burden, I'm due at the local courthouse. One of my business suppliers is suing me for supposed money owed. Dad, a retired judge, accompanies me for moral support. We share a few skittish laughs while he briefs me on how I need to lead with the judge—with truth. Based on my character evaluation of the supplier, I bet Dad $10 he will be a no show. The judge and I wait for a period of time and then the case is dismissed as he doesn't show. She asks if I want damages awarded, which I don't, though could certainly use the cash. He has enough troubles to bear by the looks of things, so I'm not going to do to him what he did to me—this wouldn't be a cool gesture.

I need to keep money flowing while I scramble to heal even though I won't push. I convince my 72-year young Dad to co-navigate a neighborhood paper route with me. It's an emotional salvation of sorts as: it only requires four hours, three times weekly; it's physically demanding, so strengthens the chest muscle cut in surgery; it allows freedom during the day to dream up what's next; it humbles me, so more quiet power is acquired; it temporarily lifts the burden of responsibility to achieve—such a relief; it offers me a priceless gem, knowing Dad in new ways—he lives without judgment and sports one wicked throwing arm; it is effortless and doesn't drain my brain—I listen to my iPod with the only pressure being to sort, stuff inserts, box papers, load the car and deliver within a three-hour window; it's routine, which creates a productive diversion, slowly drawing me out from loss—I do well with routine. We are bestowed *newspaper carrier of the month*—there is much pride in having achieved this with Dad. It is a humbling experience to say the least and my character worth has grown ten-fold.

A dear pal asks if I feel lonely. I tell her I feel alone in my situation, but not lonely.

Anger is my constant companion as impatience to get on with something threatens my *no push* default mechanism. Impatience turns into blah. I know the need to get moving, though I can't in the old ways of before. I get angry over this, but an innate wisdom, vitalheart voice won't let me pass go on any *make it happen* bus.

A close pal recently watched the movie, *The Upside of Anger;* the closing monologue is timely and profound.

> Anger and resentment can stop you in your tracks. It needs nothing to burn but the air and the life that it swallows and smothers. It's real though, the fury. Even when it isn't, it can change you, turn you, mold you and shape you into someone you're not. The upside of anger then is the person you become. Hopefully, someone that wakes up one day and realizes they are not afraid of its journey, someone who knows that the truth is, at best, a partially told story. That anger, like growth, comes in spurts and fits, and in its wake leaves a new chance at acceptance and the promise of calm.

I make myself sift through the pile of unread *Fast Company* magazines delivered monthly until the subscription runs out this December. I cherry pick one issue profiling various CEOs who recreate their lives after significant turbulence. The rest are tossed into recycling with absolutely no interest or mind for business.

The article's take-away nugget is that trauma consists of four stages: shock and disbelief; developing awareness of the loss that creates feelings of emptiness, frustration, anguish and despair (that was me six months ago); restitution—in this stage, various rituals associated with loss within a culture are performed (loss of Audi, loss of socializing due to financial constraints, loss of purchase power, loss of rapport with business contacts, loss of inclusion in circles of influence); resolution of loss—the concept of loss is idealized and preoccupation with loss gradually decreases over a year or more (that means, anytime now I may start feeling like the past is in the past); recovery—obsession with loss has ended and the individual is able to go on with his or her life.

It is said grieving takes a year.

· · · · · · · · · · ·

What imprints will I make now to create my future ideal?

My aspirations in celebrating the one-year surgery mark are primal. A focus to get out of moment-to-moment survival mode and reestablish a sense of order and safety physically, emotionally and financially is number one. Secondly, reestablishing an innate sense of safety and trust is paramount while keeping things light-hearted.

A raw vulnerability is still predominant daily. I'm not comfortable with it or the absence of inherent physical safety. I need to catch myself when I resist *what is*. To trust in new imprints, which dissolve fear over time, will transform my current relationship with uncertainty. Uncertainty can be the stepping stone to clarity and newness.

I struggle in a way never experienced before with a severely bruised sense of self. The struggle is in wrapping my head around how something like this transpired to one so athletic and health conscious. *What you resist will persist.* So, I reframe it by claiming that my strong health is what saved me. Humbling describes this past year. I notice dramatic shifts in my daily routine, unable to keep up with how differently I do things now. It's as though someone else inhabited my body with new automated ways. It's time to temper my ridiculous sense of responsibility in this second chance to live, for it weighs too heavily on me. I can choose to leave purgatory at the door!

My bravery comes and goes. When brave:

- I'm able to witness my growth with deep reverence.

- I allow myself to feel haunted.

- I practice graciousness versus resistance with a knowing that resolve of my demons is in sight.

- I engage in the most emotionally joyful moments of love from others—precious in its individual delivery.

- I've explored the strength of my spirit—understanding it can break, but never ceases to exist.

- I've evolved through many moments of sheer terror, soul-wrenching sadness and confused uncertainty from too much loss with a capacity to feel it all, and survived.

When not brave, I want to do just about anything to get outside the feelings ruling my body, mind and spirit. However, my responsibility for this second chance begs perseverance through overwhelm. The universal energy disguised as responsibility in me, which resides in each of us, prods me along. It asks that we reach outside self to serve others with innate purpose. The truth is I need to cultivate an internal purpose for external delivery.

This subtle energy is transformative in moment-to-moment living. There is richness to my stronger, quiet empowered way. Owning one's potential is an ongoing endeavor of aspiration, engagement, action and trust in uncertainty. The uncertainty begs for internal dialogue, which, if tapped and heard through your vitalheart source, will create magical imprints for the future.

- - - - - - - - - - -

TAKE-AWAY PERSPECTIVE – SILKEN LAUMANN

My inner knowing is my greatest strength as well as my greatest frustration. Just because I "know" something doesn't mean I will follow it. Although experience has shown me that I can't outsmart what I know in my deepest self, it doesn't mean I don't try. Because sometimes that deepest knowing is pretty inconvenient. Especially when it tells you that that great opportunity isn't right. My head screams, "but it's paying good money and your taxes are due." It tells me that the man I have met isn't trustworthy, even if he seems so sincere. Time after time though, knowing has led me to my True North. The inner knowing I have followed upon meeting my fiancée for the first time and coming home that night to share with a friend, "I have met the man I am going to spend the rest of my life with."

"What" she screamed! That inner knowing led me to keep pushing to uncover that my daughter wasn't a slow reader; she has a significant auditory processing challenge. That knowing leads most of the minor and major decisions I make everyday. And when something really doesn't feel right, it isn't right, no matter how good it looks, when my gut says turn around, run away, I start running. Recently I turned down a lucrative business proposal because it didn't "feel right"; just when I began to question whether I was becoming a tad flaky I learned the owner of the company had pulled up the stakes and left the country amidst noises of illegal business.

All of my work life is led by what I want to do, what I have a calling to and a passion for. I simply can't operate any other way. What I have discovered is that when you are true to this way of living your life, opportunities begin to present themselves. Christine Monaghan is an example of this in her vision of past and current endeavors. When we follow our inner knowing, chances are, things will be exactly as they should be.

— Silken Laumann
Olympian, Speaker, Writer, Kid's Champion
Silken & Co Productions Ltd
office@silkenlaumann.com
www.silkenlaumann.com

vitalheart tip

Do one thing each week you're not comfortable with. It doesn't need to be a big thing; however, do it. It will progressively inspire you toward bigger things. Conquer fear.

When uncertainty arises, take the time to respect it, to trust in your ability to sort through to truth, and then trust in acting for the highest good of this truth . . . it shall set you free.

connect possibilities
body · mind · spirit · heart

INTERNET RESEARCH

Enlighten Next .... www.enlightennext.org

The Attitude Doctor .... www.attitudedoc.com

READ

The Game of Life And How to Play It
by Florence Scovel Shinn .... www.amazon.com

The Secret of the Shadow
by Debbie Ford .... www.amazon.com

Writing Down the Bones
by Natalie Goldberg .... www.amazon.com

RENT

Dr. Seuss's Cat in the Hat......................... Video store

The Polar Express............................... Video store

DO

The Running Room .... www.runningroom.com

chapter 7
what you resist persists

"Shit happens!" the woman psychotherapist who counsels me states. She relays how imperative it is to differentiate between a specific circumstance...which one contributes to and when to practice acceptance for that which cannot be explained or assigned responsibility to. It is a slippery slope in choosing to take on shame or blame in a scenario where acceptance is needed for *what is*. When shame or blame is initiated, it translates into fear, anxiety and unhealthy obligation for self or others. It is the stuff HeartBroke spirits are made of. Suffering persists when resistance denies the gifts within *what is*.

Idiopathic is defined in Wikipedia as "an adjective used primarily in medicine meaning arising spontaneously or from an obscure or unknown cause. For most medical conditions, one or more causes are somewhat understood, but in a certain percentage of people with the condition, the cause may not be readily apparent or characterized. In these cases, the origin of the condition is said to be 'idiopathic.'"

It's probably in my best emotional interest to accept the term Idiopathic. The doctors gave this terminology as the reason for the electrical short within my heart and need for the pacemaker. I resist this inconclusive evidence with no acceptance for *what is*.

Internal rumblings churn. Further inquiry rises to the surface as the winter chill swirls outside. I ponder if we human beings actually manifest all that happens in our life, good or otherwise. This question is a given for those who've experienced a life-threatening event. What I know is that in answering this type of inquiry with an absolute yes, it means 100 percent ownership for what is or is not showing up in one's life.

The truth is I resist the notion that I created the circumstances for the need of the pacemaker. It seems preposterous to comprehend that on some level I created this experience in pursuit of the ideal. Shame and blame kick in as I wrestle between taking responsibility and surrendering to acceptance for needing the pacemaker. As I try to bounce back, I seek the learning in what did and is showing up for me.

Shame and blame are predictable emotions that show up when a major crisis or event lands on one's doorstep. More time than is healthy has been dedicated to analyzing the truth of *why* in relation to the pacemaker over the last 15 months. I do think I co-created *the crumble* events because I pushed too hard for too long. Nothing short of a significant event such as the pacemaker surgery would have slowed me down enough to take stock of the incongruent imbalance lived. However, I believe that there was something congenital going on, which was triggered by the circumstances at that point in my life. I had experienced dizziness over the past 15 years, which was diagnosed as anxiety and low blood sugar. So, it's my belief that predisposition for a negative event can exist, and then our individual experiences, beliefs and actions precipitate what takes place next.

Nourishing my spirit by surrendering resistance to know the why of the pacemaker is a practice in trusting my vitalheart source, intuition. Patience is being cultivated as I search for clarity of my truth relating to my need for a pacemaker. Patience has never been my strong suit. In the meantime, spirited learning to breathe in renewed life, vitality and clarity, through a yoga and meditation practice, occupies my time and dulls the internal chatter.

From a psychological perspective, I utilize a new technique, which is best explained as a subconscious mind re-education system, SEED (Self Empowerment Everyday). It helps transform negative, deceptive emotions and beliefs that hold one prisoner if not dealt with. The areas I hone in on with SEED are to: inch away from my shame-blame struggle and toward acceptance in my need for a pacemaker; inch forward with hope that resources to manifest healing to the degree that the pacemaker is no longer required is in my realm of possibility; inch away from dwelling on the financial debacle and make space for fresh possibilities.

* * * * * * * * * * *

If I trust the notion of manifesting all that occurs in my life, then Pippi is positive evidence of trusting in the riches received when reaching out to help another.

"What is it . . . that *s*omething that you are looking forward to?" Pippi asks in context to my possibilities and dreams beyond healing the remaining Heart*B*roke particles.

Pippi is nicknamed so for the thigh-high patterned socks she sports, which resemble Pippi Long Stockings and complement her unique way. She has become a fixture in my life the past few months and exemplifies the power of intention. Upon my business coaches' suggestion, I created a future life collage with images from magazines. One future image was adopting or mentoring a youth.

Pippi is a 16-year girl who arrived in Vancouver from Australia at Christmas time. She and her uncle Robin, my Thai masseuse friend, dropped in for a visit. We quickly formed a bond best defined as an older sister mentor, which emotionally lifts both our spirits. She struggles with an eating disorder. Pippi's family reside in Australia and, over time, her mom and I have become good pals from afar, while her uncle and a core group of friends create a safe, routine haven for her to heal. Pippi, like me with my pacemaker, will eventually need to choose exploring the underlying unknown contributors to her suffering. The collective mission is to help her to help herself.

Our defining moment of commitment to one another transpires outside Starbucks one winter afternoon where we meet after she telephones for help. I explain that my energy is limited given everything that has taken place recently. Recent wisdom encourages me to be fiercely selective in expending energy, so I will only commit to being present for her if she truly wants to live another way. Her presence more than her words reflect her want for a better way. I witness someone completely alone in a struggle and, therefore, I am unable to walk away knowing at the very least I have love to offer. So, with a mutual pact made, our worlds merge.

The following summer she moves into the suite portion of my home. Her uncle and I share legal guardianship for her until she turns 18, and our lives are forever enriched. Pippi's youthful love for all that is possible rubs off on me. I'm inspired by this new someone—Pippi! By shifting energies off my woes and toward serving another, a renewed sense of purpose is rewarded.

With a renewed sense of purpose, a quiet momentum to manifest the ideal future bubbles with cautious excitement. I want to live with purpose so I may positively impact others beyond my own wants. Capturing a child-like thrill with new possibilities for myself and those surrounded is the experience to manifest. Children are thrilled at mere thoughts of new possibilities in a moment's notice, screeching in wild abandonment in pursuit of the next experience. This type of energy is brilliant. Those who witness it in adults invariably ask, "What is it about her that she exudes such vibrancy and verve for life? I believe this sort of vibrancy comes from truly serving others from a place of passion which nurtures everyone's spirit.

I do feel a child-like thrill when my influence and energy directly benefits Pippi. It just so happens that my soul benefits as well, with priceless, intangible rewards.

* * * * * * * * * *

My hopes are disguised in small comforts that symbolize future possibilities, which I permit, despite myself.

Hope is embedded in simple comforts. I absorb the astounding beauty in the cherry blossom trees while running. I soak in the freshly-aired down quilt scent, breathing in summer. Indulging in comfort foods such as broiled tomatoes, cheese, sea salt on fresh rosemary bread with homemade tomato soup and piping hot honey tea is heart-warming soul food. My sister's familiar voice, though 3,000 miles away, reinforces how connected our hearts are. While listening to Jack Johnson, I let my mind rest with ease, enjoying his melodic tunes. Watching Rudi's ecstatic joyful hip hop from one paw to another when the treat bag appears reminds me of how the present moment is simply the best. I catch myself smiling more often.

Expectations attached to hope can take some of the comfort out of the equation though. In the past, my hopes were loaded up with detailed outcomes. Today, I practice more detachment in the final outcome, so the moment-to-moment gems are not overlooked.

Hope requires present-moment awareness for gifts not yet envisioned while practicing the law of detachment. In the past, lofty expectations tripped me up, confusing hope and expectation. In truth, what I perceived was hope were expectations for a defined outcome. When expectations are in check, marvelous new circumstances surface. When I resist *what is*, and try to control an outcome, strife tends to manifest in some way, shape or form.

Indulging in daily, simple comforts cultivates my hope. Tidbits of peace result when partaking in these comforts of choice. Though simple, they represent the future reality, a taste for what is hoped for in the grander scheme of things.

Vision is the next step once feelings of hope are activated. I'm not one for New Year's resolutions but a huge advocate of goal setting each fall. My collage symbolizes hope in new possibilities. My hope is living in this activated state of ease as the norm versus the exception. This assumes emotional, physical, financial and spiritual abundance for self, family, friends and colleagues. As trust increases through consciously indulging in small comforts, ease is spotted more frequently.

* * * * * * * * * *

An air bubble is the term used to describe what feels like trapped air in my tummy. This uncomfortable sensation is new since my surgery and best relieved with a sizable belch, which is also new to my repertoire. It takes conscious breathing in and out to belch, which can be problematic when socializing. I sense this is resistance to the pacemaker, a residual trauma of the event. The air bubbles mostly surface when I'm stressed or working out to the point of sweating.

The pacemaker website states burping is a common side effect. However, I *know* it is triggered by unhealthy stress, so I set out to manifest something different. With a willingness to try anything to end suffering, I experience various healing modalities. Desperate to feel good again, I abandon any judgment, looking beyond conventional, Western resolves.

An energetic healer arrives with a massage table, which I lay on, but she never actually touches my body with one exception. She places a cotton swab in my belly button and chants. Kaching! A homeopathic remedy promises to rid me of emotional trauma. I take one pellet with lunch and wake up six hours later in a grovel-type stupor just in time for dinner. Kaching! A practitioner suggests acid reflux and writes a prescription, which I promptly toss out. A psychologist nets a tangible insight that seems probable. His analogy to my air bubbles is, "You are still under water."

Under water best describes the drowning feelings associated with all I contend with still. So, I begin to sit with this notion as I go about my yoga and meditation practice. I'm uncertain of what the air bubbles truly represent but feel its trapped energy of some sort. Only I can do the internal work to figure it out.

It's time to allow the waves of fear to rise up and out. Accepting the grief and pain in the unanswered *why* of needing the pacemaker dissipates fear's hold. It's exhausting and only time and trust in this ultimate uncertainty will serve me. Eventually, I get to the place of acceptance for the lessons learned from the need for the pacemaker, seeing its catalyst role in my purpose. My internal jury is still out on dependency for the rest of my life.

Shame or blame are both toxic. What shame or blame story are you hauling around? What do you need to take accountability for and what do you need to accept as *what is?* Is this worn-out story sabotaging your potential? Whenever should, would, could creep into your vocabulary, you can be sure shame or blame is close at hand.

. . . .

TAKE-AWAY PERSPECTIVE – RUTH STERN

As an entrepreneur often doing things for the first time without a net, I tend to be more in the resistance category. This can't be happening to me! Push harder! Find another way! Denial, resisting, not facing the "truth" of a situation aggravates it, complicates it, prolongs it and leaves one buried in the problem itself. However, staying connected and involved, no matter how difficult the situation may be, allows you to be present, work through it and feel more like the Observer.

If it's the journey and not the destination that's important, remember many journeys have side trips.

— Ruth Stern, President and Managing Partner
www.Colour-Revolution.com

vitalheart tip: Write a letter to your old self from your new self. Dream it up and go big with your best new self! Share and be super clear on what direction you are headed in and what you're leaving behind that no longer serves you. "What's next in your realm of possibilities . . . ?"

connect possibilities
body · mind · spirit · heart

INTERNET RESEARCH

Adam, the Healer . . . . www.dreamhealer.com

Six Seconds www.6seconds.org

READ

Rich Woman by Kim Kiyosaki . . . . www.richwoman.com

The Diamond Cutter by Geshe Michael Roach
and Lama Christie McNally . . . . www.amazon.com

*The Soul of Money: Reclaiming the Wealth
of Our Inner Resources*
by Lynne Twist. . . . . www.amazon.com

chapter 8
intuition, the vitalheart voice

Cosmic constipation occurs when we don't honor our intuition and its vital creative energy. Intuition development specialist, Cheryl Brewster, shared this terrific term with me a few years back. It's a terrific reminder to continue being courageous in trusting in my vitalheart voice, intuition.

Another year is well under way. Another truth reveals my want to be a full participant in the game of life. To a large degree, I've played the observer role the past 2½ years. This role was necessary to slow down and honestly see and feel what was and wasn't working. Now, the time has come to once again step on out with a bit of uncalculated risk and a dash of spontaneity. In not honoring my vitalheart voice pre-crumble, I pushed against internal whispers and hollers, which: strongly urged against romantic involvement with an individual; kept serving up signals of pushing too hard to succeed; warned that training for a half marathon when maxed out was not the brightest idea. So, I get it now, the value in listening to the gracious voice within.

Vitalheart voice is a key factor in the grounded state I've created for myself.

In learning the hard way of what transpires when choosing to ignore this inner wisdom, I recognize confusion as the valuable tool it is. Confusion usually indicates putting off what I intuitively know needs attention. The more I put it off, the higher probability for self-doubt and uncertainty. This increases the odds in staying stuck on the object of my confusion, perpetuating unnecessary anxiety. Intuition will continue to eke me forward. This is where trust in feeling with heart instead of thinking with only my mind enters the picture. Courage is queen!

Intuition is tricky in that it is not pragmatic, factual, tangible, practical nor comfortable. It leads you toward the new, which can create interim discomfort. Lack of trust is the greatest hurdle in connecting with one's inner grace, intuition. In coining vitalheart, I demonstrate reverence to the internal heart-based knowing, the aspect of inner direction crucial to evolvement. Immense integrity with self to believe in what can't be seen and base life-altering decisions on glimpses, senses, feelings rather than cold, hard, tangible facts is required—courage in one's integrity and trust in self.

The process of dissecting numerous mundane and complex truths has been both tedious and transforming. Slowly, the worn-out perspectives have translated into refreshed experiences with new possibilities. The process precedes lightness in step if a sideways step is taken to witness the *why* behind it, how arrival at this truth of sorts began.

Examples of my worn-out truths, which now result in healthier, balanced experiences for me, are:

- Physical activity in moderation to keep healthy without extreme push and challenge.

- Waking up with my natural alarm clock, which interestingly is around 7 a.m.—civilized.

- Starting my day with a hot mug of tea, a bowl of oatmeal and fresh fruit over the period of an hour versus swigging back a shake and flying at the computer.

- Dedicating no more than seven hours daily to my career . . . no nights, no weekends . . . period.

By surrendering to *what is*, the next logical step is to trust the inner voice and make way for the entrée of new possibilities from wisdom. When I get too consumed in *what ifs*, it's virtually impossible to hear internal wisdom. This alerts the need to go for it from empowerment instead of being threatened by the unknown. The question I ask myself is, "*Chris, what do you want your experience to be while you go through transformation and change?*" Fear is the blocker to fluid energy; courage is the remedy to fear.

The Oxford dictionary defines Theosophy as the *philosophy professing to achieve knowledge of god by direct intuition*. Another term used is *knowledge of the divine*. Theosophist Madame Blavatsky's definition of magic is "wisdom applied"—the link getting you from intuition to action where magic, wonder and awe exist. She claimed a three-pronged link: connect to and with your heart; acknowledge and celebrate the stage you are leaving; and lead in integrity and intention.

One of her maxims (general truth, rule of conduct briefly expressed) is compassion is the law of laws. She explained that brotherhood is not a mere ideal—it is a fact in nature on the spiritual plane. From that we derive a logical basis and a binding voice for morality that can guide and inspire us, even while more traditional religious voices are losing their compelling force. She gives us the *"metaphysics from which we can deduce the most important principles of how to live."* www.blavatsky.net

The current mantra of choice echoes in my head, *I'm stronger than I think I am.* Assessment for who I've become combined with manifested possibilities result in a new-found sense of ease, which I craved my entire life. I recite the mantra often while I step past comfort zones in many respects. A revitalized spirit emerges each time. This takes courage to confront the gnawing, subtle energy of residual trauma, which prevents me from completely living with ease.

Residual trauma can be insidious and hardwired on a cellular level if awareness to its cries are not met with courage and empathy. So, I practice delegating these cries to my vitalheart voice. My current need is to uncover the truth behind the pained expression my tummy discomfort now delivers up. My hunch is it represents residual trauma, current and, perhaps, long term since childhood. And, so it goes. *I am stronger than I think I am!*

Harnessing more potential through practicing the three-pronged approach is simple as far as Madame Blavatsky is concerned. My take on her theory is this: First, connect to and with your heart—the state of confusion or uncertainty diminishes when you choose making a shift based on what your heart feels. This leads to transcending the confusion into action from a place of wisdom. Second, acknowledge and celebrate the stage you have left or are leaving. Celebrate this with triggers that feel good—buy a new candle scent, eat a new food, drink something out of the ordinary, listen to new types of music. These intuitively derived experiences shift initiating from head to heart. Third, integrity and intention . . . Utilize your deliberate focus for the most beneficial and productive you by getting clear and clean on what your truth is, then trust in it.

> Three things cannot long be hidden: the sun, the moon, and the truth.
> — Confucius

• • • • • • • • • • •

Tummy troubles slowly entered my life this spring and, by the end of the year, are literally creating quite a stir. After tests and prodding from traditional and non-traditional practitioners, I get an IBS diagnosis. Irritable Bowel Syndrome is a condition that affects a huge percentage of the population, women are more susceptible. It is a digestive disorder with no known cause, another idiopathic scenario. My symptoms include tummy muscle spasms after eating, constipation and severe dizziness when it's a really bad bout.

My intuition tells me from the outset it's stress, that the residual trauma is alive and thriving in my cells. So, I stop eating wheat and dairy on the recommendation of the naturopath after food allergy tests are conducted. This results in more weight loss, of concern to not just me. I take digestive enzymes, pop acidophilus at night and begin acupuncture. The traditional doctor gives me a prescription, which I toss away. I will not be another statistic masking what the body cries out to have healed.

After a time, I know it's up to me to resolve this within. The well-intended practitioners have greatly contributed to taming the symptoms, but there is a need to re-configure some worn-out truths, negative thoughts! After all, I'm the only one in my thoughts, which I believe trigger the IBS. Since I was a kid, I remember experiencing tummy aches when eating this or that or experiencing stressful times. It's time to really claim the truth in how I process stress given an acute sensitivity to both food and interactions I witness with others.

Connecting with the Chinese medicine practitioner who applies acupuncture weekly for months is a blessing. Exercise is limited on days where a flare up makes even walking down the lane uncomfortable; and so, I practice acceptance in the moment, though I am determined this is not to going to be my new norm. If I pop some ibuprofen, it is manageable. And I pop more than I'd like to while working through *it*. Toward the end of this year, I purchased a hypnosis DVD set from a doctor in London promising relief. It complements the previous healing modalities and I'm 75 percent good most of the time. I share this crumble associated malady with only a few as it's one more thing to add to what feels like a boring sob story. Enough already!

With exercise unpredictable, I buy some power yoga DVDs. The DVDs are grace in action and become a four-times weekly ritual, which my body and spirit now crave, a delicious lifestyle shift.

No ha ha's, that's for sure. I assume my crumble learning is not done, so I get quiet and begin daily meditation with my iPod, usually in the late afternoon before dinner. It brings me calm and guidance and my spirit soaks it up. I crave it like I used to crave my afternoon Starbucks Chai Tea Latte . . . Ah, Grasshopper!

Like Dorothy clicking her glass slippers together and chanting, "There's no place like home," my most recent mantra inches me toward greater strength. *I'm stronger than I think I am.* It helps me when I'm unsure. It gives me courage in its absence.

"Are you rebuilding or simply building?" My blooming romantic interest says with wisdom less the judgment . . .

Blooming romance is in the works, one which ends my self-imposed two-year intimate lock down. His recent words make me pause. My spiel of the last 2½ years involves sharing the *hows and whys* of *rebuilding* my world. The time to shift this perspective from rebuild, as we human beings are always in build mode, is here. This shift permits me to feel whole again instead of feeling less than with the pacemaker. The fact is, it was and is always good if I choose to see it with wise eyes and an open heart. If this verbiage continues by speaking in terms of rebuild, I risk getting stuck in a story of feeling less than all I've become, crippled by circumstances instead of empowered. More begets more of the same. Conscious celebration has no room to inspire if lack is predominant. Yikes and Wow!

To *rebuild* generally infers starting from scratch, implying nothing before this point is carried forward with you. So my sweetie's wise words encourage me to reframe what story is being created now because you never really start from scratch. To *build* is: to foster momentum; to utilize my wound's essence and wins to evolve; to not push, but gently stretch myself, sometimes further than I think capable of; to not get bunged up in cosmic constipation; to trust in what's next with a positive question mark to discover unlimited potential.

The real gem from his words is this. If I truly want to own my potential, then *building* is the daily ongoing catalyst to realize it. I begin to feel the positive energy shift when I choose this perspective for moving forward, unencumbered from the thought of digging out from under. I begin to trust this new truth as life thrives again with much to be grateful for.

So, the task is to connect with my vitalheart voice where love resides and *build* from this position of empowerment with anything or anyone. Courage will carry me by feeling fear and acting despite it—moving through versus around it. Moving through fear requires staying present and venturing toward possibilities not yet considered from the place of love with an open heart. I need to keep my heart open.

What do you want to build that requires a bit or heap of courage, a resolve of fear? Who or what leads you from a place of fear versus love? Why? What is keeping you from realizing your potential due to this fear? Are you rebuilding or building?

· · · · · · · · · · ·

What's courage got to do with it?

The level of courage has everything to do with positive perspective and current truth. My conversation with Christine Brown, a meditation teacher in Vancouver, BC, is enlightening, uplifting and she is just adorable. Her insights perpetuate courage.

I believe regardless of one's spiritual or religious practices, Buddhist teachings, if practiced, go a long way to increase happiness and minimize suffering.

The Buddhist approach to resolving fear is to investigate what lurks under fear's surface, to detect the core issue. This involves courage to confront that which we would rather deny. The approach I practice is putting aside my *"self cherishing"* state of mind, my state of self-involved fear and shift my focus toward another. This shifts me into empowerment.

Cherishing is the grasping of whom or what I believe is my truth in relation to a specific fear. This delusion of sorts keeps me stuck. It is my self-imposed perception of who I believe I am in context to the fear. In Buddha terms, self-cherishing is the mental attitude where one considers self to be supremely important and precious, translating into cherishing oneself too much, creating fear. Paralysis per se is the outcome that prevents one from overcoming the fear. To let go or release grasping is to fear less and live more. I work on acknowledging fear and anger, dissolving its warped power, so it doesn't become my new story.

So, I look to sourcing a loving reason, something outside of myself when fear lurks. I test trusting love to dissolve fear. When I'm gripped by fear, anger exists in some derivative: frustration, irritation, impatience and criticism. When angry, the space isn't conducive to love or for healing to occur. No good comes from anger (fear). So, I practice patience and acceptance to counter anger (fear) by getting comfortable with things being as they are now. This healing stuff is tough work!

Buddhist teacher, Christine Brown says her flag in suffering and not living a state of belief is when: she feels heavy; she is in the *"It's all about me"* thought process; she focuses strictly on self instead of others as well. However, she stresses the importance to maintain doing things that keep YOU strong, relaxed and healthy on all levels. This gives you presence and strength of mind to lift others up. But, the all-consuming "I" is not in anyone's best interest.

My take-away from her wisdom is to consciously focus on being and doing each day with positive mindfulness of and for others as it can only transcend my relationship with self and others. My want is to step outside my self-interest, take the bloody courage pill as often as need be and start focusing on how I can elevate others.

* * * * * * * * * *

Courage in the form of listening to my vitalheart voice is presenting wonders with much gratefulness: a budding romance creates fun, love and support, along with a teen miss and pets galore; a reciprocal influence of love feeds both Pippi and I; a place I call the Sugar Shack is the oceanfront cottage I now call home; a monthly *"Own Your Potential"* column, fuels my creative spirit; an increased sense of physical strength increases trust; and a clean bill of health with the annual pacemaker checkup is comforting.

My blossoming romance is sweet, tender and makes everything seem a bit brighter, easier to handle and, well, just like we all want trusting love to feel—joyful, loving and mutually appreciative. Yes, my two-year intimate lock down is over—like riding a bicycle, you fall off and then just hop back on a new set of wheels with desire, adventure and pleasure in tow. We slowly share and merge our worlds with respect for each others' mutual need to nurture love and equality with the absence of forced obligation as a foundation.

* * * * * * * * * *

Home now resides at the Sugar Shack. Pippi and I first set foot in here in the spring. Over the last six months, I'd envisioned our home as a West Vancouver ocean cottage, so when I spot the ad in a local newspaper, I know it is ours. I turn to Pippi and say, *"This is where we heal."* The sea air is pure tonic. I finally exhale, relaxing in body, mind and spirit. This is the time and place to go within to heal core trauma. My lifestyle is healing oriented with sleep-ins, reading on the porch couch, watching the busy, ocean marine traffic, eating well and slowly to candlelight and soothing music, meandering down the lane numerous times daily with the pups, and creating community by getting to know neighbors. In general, we live a simple, yet rich existence with a pact to alleviate pressure, drama and chaos.

* * * * * * * * * *

Passion pops up into more than one area of my life. Writing for an hour feels like five minutes. Time sails by when curled under the couch duvet on the porch while writing and taking in the moving montage on the ocean. When in writing mode, I'm connected here on Earth. I realize my great fortune in figuring this piece out, this voice of connectivity on Earth. I don't want to waste this blessing—it, and I, deserve to flourish.

* * * * * * * * * *

The lead up to my third annual pacemaker checkup is easier than the previous two. Largely because my life is really good again, so I'm more gracious with the gadget. I ponder how to spend the day. It comes to me during yoga that a regular day of ease is my best experience imaginable.

The checkup involves a computer mouse placed on top of the pacemaker, and then a download of all necessary information from last year's use. Several tests are done to identify various thresholds such as battery life and high- and low-pace settings based on each patient's particular condition. For me, the pacemaker kicks in when my blood pressure goes below 60. It brings it back up and won't allow it to go below the 60 mark. One test manipulates this process to ensure the low and high thresholds are accurate. I detest this one. It triggers the exact dizziness felt when rushed to the hospital—how do you spell trauma?

Another test is equally frightening, speeding my heart rate up. I feel like I'm moving quickly, though lying still wrapped in wires and sensors, like aliens invading your body. Anxious is an understatement during these tests, leaving me vulnerable. Still pissed in needing the pacemaker, I'm angry my body can't independently function properly. Another opportunity to surrender to the premise, *it is what it is*. Acceptance isn't achieved yet, so gentle courage is needed.

An interesting statistic from this checkup is my body is only using the pacemaker 86 percent versus 98 percent of the time in one year. I've believed since day one that if I can access an innate ability to heal myself, one day I will no longer need it. My pact is to focus on this belief nightly when tucked into bed. My hope is to energetically alter things so my body's electrical system becomes 100 percent functional on its own.

So, what's next? Next is to feel like a full participant in the game of life on my own terms instead of a spectator watching from the sidelines. This sense of sitting on the sidelines the past three years feels like a forced containment of my own doing. Neutral is the predominant emotional state I've created, a protection from chaos and stress, which

I have no desire to handle, but I may have gone a bit far in this pursuit. I wouldn't do it differently if given another chance. This provokes me to inch out of my comfort zone by focusing on: being the best mentor possible for Pippi by thriving in my life; being a positive influence and friend to the teen miss, my sweetie's daughter; being a voice of love, strength, wisdom and inspiration for my sweetie; and being my own best friend with constant shifts to positive perspectives by honoring truth and trusting in my process.

My last words on ensuring regularity from cosmic constipation are:

- Don't resist your intuitive feelings.

- Act upon these feelings with full trust in your innate ability to know the right way for you.

- Trust yourself (your intuitions) enough to know the next right thing to do.

- Follow through even when present circumstances (and even future) don't appear aligned or practical.

- Surrender to the possibility of the result taking you out of your *comfortableness* toward something that isn't guaranteed.

* * * * * * * * * * *

If you tell a lot of fibs externally, your internal dialogue will generally reflect the same inconsistency. It's hard to get a grip on your personal power and realize your full potential as a spiritual being about

yourself if highly inaccurate or if you constantly buy the ego's story and head up the wrong path.

— Stuart Wilde

. . . .

TAKE-AWAY PERSPECTIVE – CHERYL BREWSTER

How do we translate those chronic, gnawing feelings of knowing that something is off-kilter, yet not knowing why, what "it" is or how to fix it? Do we tend to put more pressure on ourselves to feel better, do better, accomplish more, or on the opposite side of the spectrum, go into total denial, living zombie-like because it hurts too much to do otherwise?

Being kind to ourselves in the process of discovery is the Higher Self's wisdom—guiding us back to our brilliance, the intuitive flow that releases our creative urges so they are birthed, grounded and effective. How brave we are in our truth journeys, and how important that we share our stories with each other, for in that sharing we experience the meaning and value of our very selves, and that we are not alone. Sometimes the most daring thing we can do is surrender, to follow that forbidden call to honor the needs of the self, and say, "I see you, and I am committed to honoring what you need." The discomfort in our bodies, emotions and minds are wake-up calls, signals, beeps, alarms that get our attention. Vitalheart voice moves within us for a reason—it can be trusted, in being willing to give up the lives we knew, we discover the one we were truly born to live. That's truth—that's intuition—that's vitalheart voice.

— Cheryl Brewster
Professional Clairvoyant, Speaker, Intuition Development Specialist
www.theintuitivelife.com

vitalheart tip — Get quiet with yourself. Even if for only 10 minutes a day while driving to and from. Choose something of focus that you want clarity on, then ask a question and be quiet. Keep going back to the question each day for as much time as you think you deserve to receive the answer. You will be amazed at what surfaces.

connect possibilities
body · mind · spirit · heart

INTERNET RESEARCH

Help for IBS . . . . www.helpforibs.com

Michael Mahoney Hypnosis CDs . . . .
www.michaelmahoneyhypnotherapist.com

Theosophist Madame Helena
Blavatsky's . . . . www.blavatsky.net

New York Insight Meditation Centre . . . . . www.nyimc.com

David Hamann . . . . www.coachingfrominside.com

READ

Laws of Success by Napoleon Hill . . . . . . www.amazon.com

The E-Myth Revisited by Michael Gerber . . . .
www.amazon.com

The Power of Full Engagement
by Jim Loehr and Tony Schwartz . . . . . . www.amazon.com

The Seven Spiritual Laws of Success
by Deepak Chopra . . . . www.chopra.com

LISTEN

Doreen Virtue Meditations . . . . www.angeltherapy.com

DO

Chinese Medicine (acupuncture) . . . . . . www.tazoodle.com

chapter 9
p.s. i love you

♡ Love heals the wound it makes.

— Eva Cassidy

Conceal in fear or reveal with love? A new year beginning with transitions realized, all fueled by love since *the crumble* four years ago. This love is about owning my power once again by delivering refreshed truths and trusting in the process of where it will take me. Passion has returned from living my truth from this place of love.

In experiencing positive evidence of *what is*, created from a state of love instead of fear, my level of trust in truth strengthens, a habit, requiring less conscious attention. This love has transformed numerous parts of my life. I now share legal guardianship of Pippi with her uncle. My romance becomes more entwined with a sense of voluntary belonging, making everything more pleasurable. The abrupt end to a career project contract provokes freedom to get real about my potential. Passion returns as I listen to the intuitive murmurs of heart in harmony with my pragmatic mind. Dreams begin to unfold as my perspective shifts from utter loss of trust in body, mind and spirit to renewed understanding of my innate power source, the vitalheart voice.

The litmus test of current evolvement with truth is in recognizing my hard edge, which attempts to protect me. However, it literally squashes the soft, innate trust as my spirit of voice, muscles and heart tighten. It awakens me to the fact of denial in truth as fear surfaces. I believe the most debilitating fear is the one(s) we masterfully conceal from others. The attempt to convince ourselves that *it* is not making us small, and our denial of *it* keeps us confined from trusting in truth. It mirrors our level of current value for self.

If I want to yield a surplus of abundance in my life, then I need only to remember to act from love for self and others, period. This developing love for self has pulled me through a very dark period of time. How ironic that the single most crippling state any of us can engage in is fear. It sucks the very life and love out of individuals, denying the giving or receiving of the very thing they struggle to attain—love.

A Dorothy Thompson quote speaks to this notion, *"There is nothing to fear except the persistent refusal to find out the truth, the persistent refusal to analyze the causes of happenings."*

· · · · · · · · · · · ·

♡ I believe that unarmed truth and unconditional love will have the final word in reality. This is why right, temporarily defeated, is stronger than evil triumphant.

— Martin Luther King

. . . .

Love gets concealed by fear. Fear certainly took its best shot to make me small over the years with a tremendous cost, like *the crumble*. If I had lead from truth instead of being driven by fear, I may have made different choices prior to *the crumble*. And though I still may have required the pacemaker, I'd have surrendered to a lot of things way before being forced to. I just kept on going out of fear of my life collapsing. And, it did anyway. In concealing fear pre- and post-crumble, I endured more suffering than needed, isolated myself, prolonged healing, suffered needless exhaustion, plus caused pain and disappointment from others toward me by not trusting enough to reveal *it*, my truth.

Irrational fear and old habits really didn't want out of the picture; however, my mission for a healthier way possessed a stronger, more authentic conviction, so, eventually tamed the beast a great deal.

My experience with irrational fear is it minimizes one's peace due to *what ifs* instead of the very useful, instinctive mechanism, intuition, which protects me from stepping off the curb into oncoming traffic. Not a day goes by that I don't wrestle irrational fear by willing love's dominance to strengthen me. Irrational fear has been a real struggle since *the crumble*, temporarily crippling me as I concealed its power over me to others. I concealed it to save face with others so they wouldn't worry about me. I wanted to appear stronger than I was, trying to convince myself that functionality wasn't impeded. I concealed it, thinking the internal terror might dissipate if I denied its existence. I concealed it to fulfill responsibility for this second crack at life. Mostly, I concealed it to deny any residual trauma, falsifying a sense of being healed. The truth was, and is, *the crumble* took me to my knees and I'm learning a new definition of strength by being vulnerable.

Old habits die hard. Fear is my oldest, crippling habit that keeps me contained, less than I can become. The recent paralyzing fear from my crumble cost me dearly. I missed a dear friend's wedding because I emotionally couldn't deal with traveling and, financially, had not a dime to spare given business-related repayment commitments. Another friendship was tarnished when I opted out of speaking at her mom's funeral—I was still too raw to handle being that strong for another. Fear cost me a potentially amazing career opportunity of traveling the world on private jets and yachts as the personal assistant to one of Canada's most elite businessmen. It seemed incongruent and too overwhelming at the time. It cost me going to a Christina Aguilera concert—Pippi got concert tickets for my birthday, and on the day of I couldn't handle the crowds and didn't have even $10 extra cash to get there, back or dine out. The truth is I disappointed these individuals in the moment, but I was finally beginning to trust listening to what Chrissie needed first.

Though it appears irrational fear has held me captive, the reality is that my love of self is starting to work its magic. At first glance, these choices look like avoidance, however, a non-negotiable pact to self is teaching me to nurture self first with a responsibility to others second. It has felt enormously uncomfortable and self-involved. It's been the source of significant confusion and angst, such a departure from the person I formerly was. The choices have all been good ones, though tough to make. This has taken immense strength to go against the grain of what is considered acceptable.

The biggest hurdle to overcome is a tremendous disappointment in my former self and confusion with this new self. It has taken a lot of love to trust a new way, which is so polarized. The former Chrissie never missed out on an opportunity to share in a new experience. I felt extreme fear in allowing less than, and accepted my choices with great resistance at the time, which made for buckets of tears and sadness of the price paid during *the crumble* fallout. I let pride get the better of me when I didn't reveal my current truth because the Chrissie pre-crumble would have rallied, thrived and taken initiative to make it all happen. I now get how this perspective was off and my choices were correct in the moment. I'm deeply sorry for those negatively affected by these choices. It does not reflect my love for you, rather my need to utilize love to resolve my own fear.

Excuses for containing one's fear in order to conceal the truth only leads to pain for all involved. The amount of energy that fancy footwork takes to conceal subtly seeps into every inch of our being to keep us small. It limits liberation. When justifying *just one more time*, it permits resistance to truth. This blocks change with no space for freedom to thrive. Untapped potential is left on the curb, by us. Just one more time leads to crisis mode bit by bit. Bewildered, frustrated and paralyzed with fear leaves no room for an iota of peace. This batters and weakens our system creating an unhealthy, perpetual cycle of vulnerability, which stunts our sense of self—physically, emotionally, financially, spiritually and intellectually.

The hidden gift in revealing one's truth with another exists in the possibility for equal reciprocation for pure authenticity. I am learning to take the focus off how others will perceive and respond to the truth, as it only stifles our respective voices and contributes to a collective smallness of character. Sometimes, voices differ vastly and this is not bad. Agreeing to disagree is healthy as long as one is ever so mindful of not trashing someone in the process. It takes a great deal more courage to be truthful from the outset when you know the other party will be opposed, but put it out there anyway because you are trusting in the concept of truth and love conquers all. It is the greatest demonstration of love, respect and value for self and towards others.

. . . .

♡ **Impersonal Love**
Even after all this time,
The sun never says to the earth, "You owe me."
Look what happens with a love like that – it lights the whole sky

— Hafiz

. . . .

What would love do now?

In my view, the contrast to fear is love. The question, *what would love do now*, has been useful when I need to confront a fear or negative circumstance. It raises my awareness and shifts my energy to come at fear from a positive perspective. This positively influences the desired outcome and ekes me away from negative thoughts.

This notion is based on trying to take the high road in situations when negative or challenging elements exists. It leads to compassion when anger, fear and impatience want to settle in. It gives me the opportunity to be gracious and respond instead of react to unpleasantness. It ups my ante to lead as I would like to follow, with respect and consideration for others. It softens the potential for conflict by managing a difference of opinion between loved ones in a gentle manner, reigning in harshness.

To live this way takes ongoing practice, which consistently tests me. I know when I come from this place because I frequently enjoy fun. More energy is freed up to nurture self and others. I soften with ease. Critical judgments are few and far between. Productivity is more effortless and purposeful. When another reacts by lashing out at my truth, though I don't appreciate their tone, I accept it as their perspective and try simply to move on instead of stooping down by engaging in a spitting match.

Trusting represents approaching my life from a state of love versus fear. The more I trust, the more I build love for self. This perpetuates acting from truth and a greater love for self ensues. It's just as easy to extend a warm hand as a cold one. The difference being, a hand of warmth feeds both individuals whereas the hand of coldness chills both.

* * * * * * * * * *

As a seeker of my truth, I'm consciously choosing to be accountable by being mindful and aware. It is the only way through muck and the most efficient way to touch the next best thing.

Recently, I spoke my truth in a business environment. I knew that in doing so, I was forcing so-called superiors into accountability. However, I couldn't limp along not producing. It had become unacceptable to me to continue receiving payments for productivity that was capped due to a lack of support and information. The ongoing justifications for my not receiving guidance and resources were getting tired and my credibility was at stake, mostly to myself. The environment was highly charged with political agendas, though my only agenda was to do the best job possible.

I had repeatedly expressed to the leaders not feeling good about a lack of information and support, which I stated was minimizing my potential. My tummy was in knots with the lack of response, actions and concern. So, in a last-ditch attempt to utilize my atrophying skills, I ruffled a few feathers to garner some much needed action. I gave them more credit for a stronger sense of self than to literally set me free the following day with no cause per se. I hadn't anticipated that in speaking my truth, I'd get hung out to dry by the very ones who preached being my biggest advocates. I had been played by some of these advocates who had repeatedly agreed that challenges existed that minimized my ability to succeed. Now it was clear that transparent communication was not entirely welcomed.

This experience netted terrific lessons. It is not what one says, but what one actually does that determines a perception of their leadership acumen. My ideal environment for optimum productivity, purpose and profit starts with the coexistence of truth and accountability for and with one another. If this means requesting another to be accountable for what is or is not taking place under their lead, then so be it. The leaders I want to work in tandem with are willing to hear all sides, are willing to acknowledge when different perspectives just might be of value versus a threat to the herd mentality.

This experience reinforced that politics tend to be a fear-based phenomena and mostly toxic cultures, which thrive and sustain themselves on hierarchy through fear. Fortunately, I've developed a strong enough sense of self to know that I can't thrive or function in such an environment. I get that I can have all the grand intentions, energy, skill set and resources to be wildly successful for the benefit of others, but if not reciprocated, then it is a waste of everyone's time and money—in this case, the tax payers.

The take-away for me is to make sure I lead as I would like to follow given I'd just experienced the flipside of this premise. Suffice to say, spirit of truth in leadership isn't what first pops in my head at the mention of individuals who were supposedly guiding me. It's all good, just not the environment I wish to be associated with or influenced by. I'm sure they were relieved to have this truth seeker out of their hair as well. I'm proud of the strength I showed and, given the chance to do it again, I would only change one thing . . . I'd thank them for showing me how not to lead with others.

With nothing but time on my side after this project ending, I came to realize there's no time like now to build my own thing again. In coming full circle in four years to create another business focusing on the riches in health, a pride prevails. It's the mere start of a new chapter in my story!

The thing is, sharing truth can be messy in the moment, but it is the surest way to the next best thing for all concerned. As Dad says, "War rules, love conquers." You can always choose where to lead from. You simply decide to practice moving through fear toward truth with love and compassion for self as situations drudge up the garbage. Let fear be your signpost of potential untapped, awaiting your attention.

Pick one small fear you've concealed away. Trust sharing it with one you love and notice how tightness melts away and love envelops. Dare another to glimpse at their fear to witness liberation by love. I think William Sloane Coffin's quote speaks to my perspective well. "The world is too dangerous for anything but truth and too small for anything but love."

> ♡ All schools, all colleges, have two great functions: to confer, and to conceal, valuable knowledge. The theological knowledge which they conceal cannot justly be regarded as less valuable than that which they reveal. That is, when a man is buying a basket of strawberries it can profit him to know that the bottom half of it is rotten.
> — Mark Twain

> ♡ It's just a ride. And we can change it anytime we want. It's only a choice. No effort, no work, no job, no savings of money. A choice, right now, between fear and love. The eyes of fear want you to put bigger locks on your door, buy guns, close yourself off. The eyes of love, instead, see all of us as one.
> — Bill Hicks

. . . .

TAKE-AWAY PERSPECTIVE – FAWN CHRISTENSON

Christine has tapped in to the pulse of love returning to our awareness. Continuing to trust one's self and one's truth allows the flow of love to be present between the people and events taking place. In her journey, of trusting and then speaking her truth, the love and nurturing process had become palpable. From her experiences we can see for ourselves how this process allows what is best for our well-being to happen. Once again, her courage models to us all that choosing life from a state of love versus fear is always worth it.

I applaud Christine's message of "putting myself first in the nurturing process with a responsibility to others second." Can we relearn our own value through love? What if we all opened to forgiveness of ourselves, allowing love to return to our awareness? Could we all then see and experience a world of peace and safety and joy? Let us be inspired by Christine's voice and trust our own hearts in guiding ourselves to act from our truth.

— Fawn Christianson
Fawn@FawnC.com
www.connecttoabundance.com

vitalheart tip
Each time you catch yourself in a state of worry, anxiety or fear mode, tell it to buzz off. It is a terrific, instantaneous release and gradually minimizes its existence. Wear an elastic band on your wrist and each time you're aware of these negative ninnies, snap the band and say, "I hear you, you are safe, thank you."

connect possibilities
body · mind · spirit · heart

INTERNET RESEARCH

30-Day Writing Challenge . . www.writethedamnbook.com

College of Sexual Knowledge
and Love Coaching . . . . www.loveologyuniversisty.com

Sacred Heart Path . . . . www.sacredheartpath.com

The Journey, Brandon Bays . . . . www.thejourney.com

Uplifting Quotes. . . . . www.wisdomquotes.com

Braveheartwomen. . . . . www.braveheartwomen.com

READ

The Heart of the Healer
by Bernie Segal . . . . www.berniesegalmd.com

LISTEN

Songbird by Eva Cassidy . . . . www.amazon.com

DO

George's Aloe Vera Liquid . . . . . . www.warrenlabsaloe.com

Power Yoga for Happiness . . . . www.eoinfinnyoga.com

Ali McGraw: Yoga, Mind and Body . . . . .www.amazon.ca

chapter 10
uncertainty & the global heart

♡ Be patient toward all that is unsolved in your heart.
And try to love the questions themselves.
— Rainer Maria Rilke

Uncertainty. I only recently uncovered the wisdom in uncertainty as the incredible gift intended for my life. It politely suggests creating space within to access my vitalheart, to guide toward a refreshed truth. My learning is that when in a state of uncertainty, it usually indicates that I'm not trusting in my truth, so not acting in respect of it, or I'm not certain what the current truth is. Not trusting in it or acting in respect of it is simply about not honoring my worth. Being uncertain of what the truth is indicates that a shift in perspective is on the horizon, one that better serves me now. New possibilities are endless if I choose to trust exploring.

It makes sense now, that quiet voice that beckoned me to write a book as I lay on the ER gurney five years ago, on October 1st. At that point in time, I innately knew to trust in my vitalheart voice. Recently, I became clear in the hidden, healing gem for writing this book. The gem is uncertainty, and its role played, spanning from childhood to present. Uncertainty is that *thing* for me, the *thing* I've struggled with in this lifetime in too many forms to mention.

This *thing* is different for everyone; however, I'm pretty sure uncertainty is a stressor for many. It's the part of our story that plays out as suffering time and time again, until we finally identify and acknowledge it, surrender and befriend it. Then, we can consciously choose to shift our perspective in relationship to it. With awareness, attention and true commitment, it can become our greatest gift to self and others. Uncertainty nudges me to tap into my vitalheart voice and gain clarity. Who would of thunk?

Throughout the past five HeartBroke years since *the crumble,* I frequently doubted myself for the time taken to earnestly feel wholehearted and vibrant again. Questioning why it was taking so bloody long, I wondered how many more lessons were coming down the pike until a place of constant ease and acceptance could be the norm. Patience, Grasshopper! It has taken the time it did, so once and for all, I can befriend a life-long burden. This subtle, destructive burden of angst was masked as *anxiety, worry, push to make it happen and impatience,* all to stave off uncertainty. True peace eluded me as a friction to coexist with such a strong force of denial, and resistance was hard at work, fighting for dominance. WOW and Yikes!

These writings and innate, magical findings have provided a safe and humbling place to once again ignite my sparkle. A growing certainty builds within, each time I listen to my vitalheart and trust in *a* given truth. A connected sense of ease, possibility and confidence in leading from truth continues to present amazing individuals and circumstances into my world that are truly vital.

> ♡ Men stumble over the truth from time to time, but most pick themselves up and hurry off as if nothing happened.
> — Winston Churchill

. . . .

AM I STILL HEARTBROKE?

Gratefully, I've paced through *the crumble* with an open, vital heart full of love and reverence. Halleluiah! In wading through the muck, I gradually chose to author a refreshed story. I suppose this choice represented a belief in universal love and happenstance. I just knew I wasn't intended to experience all the incredible and not so incredible things to settle out in mediocrity.

We each have an emotionally charged story we've created: one based on our actual experiences from choices made; one based on how we've chosen to perceive these experiences; and one that's created perceptions moving us closer to or farther away from untapped potential.

For me, mending my Heart*B*roke state has come down to progressively shifting my many perceptions, which created severe uncertainty from *the crumble* circumstances and the time leading up to it. Just now, I can articulate it as such, though instinctively, I was growing through old, worn-out beliefs without consciously connecting the dots as such until now. As I continue to consciously influence my evolving story, I will focus on being helpful and contribute to others in all that I do and be. I will share my experiences, learning, resources and tools in hopes that they too will consider exploring what their truth is from the mundane to the complex by trusting in their own vitalheart.

Uncertainty and change are constant—halves of the same whole. So, this is where most would rewind to childhood and identify the circumstances leading to nasty and persistent adult shortcomings. My childhood was mostly loving, full and healthy. My parents did the best they knew how. And, though a *Monaghan story exists* like most families worldwide, at some point I chose to carry the good forward after reconciling what didn't work with my unique self. My parents have always encouraged us to go for it, to explore what our interests are. This has given me a strong sense of self, the greatest gift a parent can instill in their children. Thank you, Mum and Dad, for this most precious gift.

> ♡ Would we humans know our heart in truth, nothing on earth would be impossible for us.
> — Paracelsus

. . . .

So, here goes my childhood truth. Uncertainty was plenty even though our upper-middle-class family didn't go without vacations, a home half a block from the beach, tennis clubs, and indulgence in many parties and hobbies. We laughed lots, spent many summer nights having picnics at the beach. Mum and Dad were our biggest fans. They showed up and cheered us on at sports events followed by an ice cream stop. I loved my Mary Poppins room, complete with matching curtains, bedspread and wall paper. They indulged the kids in the neighborhood when we put on dress-up fashion shows in the garden while they sipped their summer G&Ts. I still try to emulate the feel of Sunday nights with roast beef, Yorkshire pudding, steam pudding and hot custard. This was followed by tucking into clean, air-dried sheets for a dreamy sleep. I witnessed much affection between my parents and remember their hugs, kisses and guffawing.

And, our family experienced its share of crisis, loss and dysfunction. My overly sensitive nature spent too much time concerned with everyone else's *stuff*. I didn't know how to detach from fixing other's pain, so became a pretty good problem solver. The other kids in the neighborhood seemed to scamper about without a care in the world. I was clueless in handling the intensity of emotions harbored on behalf of others, so stuffed most away knowing sharing them rattled others' comfort zones. I was overly responsible with those I loved, so a premature seriousness consumed me—I took on the weight of the world, but few knew.

Energy was divided between sopping up solo time and being a social butterfly depending on what scene was playing out at home. At an early age, I experienced an acute sense of knowing in others, of what the real deal was, my intuition was alive and thriving. To a degree, I buried it with teen sophistication when not knowing how to process some truths. I was spunky, feisty and spirited. Big on my priority list was enjoying fits of hysterical laughter while inadvertently acquiring bouts of wisdom well beyond my years, cultivated through observance. A Cancerian entertainer at heart, I was all about fun for the most part. Periodically, this was interrupted by a shy, reflective kid based on my mood and environmental circumstances. Physically super strong, I'm blessed to have been born into this particular family, quirks and all. They influenced who I am today. I truly like hanging with me, so I'm grateful for each of the six family members, including me. It's all good!

TODAY'S JOURNEY

One day, today, I finally know. I need to learn to trust me again, maybe truly for the first time.
I watch joggers on the seawall—that was once me daily.
But today, my tummy resists this short stroll.
A wave of sensation washes through me, not quite pain, yet a sense of impending doom should I continue is triggered within.
I detest it. I feel old, weak, prune-like, though young, vital and athletic in the eyes of any passerby.
Tears won't surface, just confusion and frustration for resolve.
Trust?—If not now, when?—If not myself, then how with others?
How is this lack of trust serving me in staying small?
Peace, purpose, productivity, strength and love—all thrive from trust.
This body served me well for 42 years, and then took a brief respite.
Perhaps I pushed it—denied or mistrusted its calls for balance.
It temporarily stopped.
It keeps me stalled emotionally for optimum physical prowess.
I beg to move effortlessly with innate trust propelling me onward.
In my eyes, I'm less than with lack of trust in body?
Compromised; flat vs. shining; incomplete, not whole; not leading in absolute truth; a bit of a lie to all, ultimately to myself.
Struggle. This silent, concealed, exhaustive fear pokes away at me.
I continually fight for normalcy in once, taken-for-granted activities.
Not living physical potential chips away at my spirit.
Polarized from running far and fast to now running away from . . .
How or what to start trusting my innate, *know-how* safety, strength and fun in the frivolous?
Just do, Chrissie! With compassion and courage when awareness hits.
Explore versus escape; do versus talk; surrender versus fight; love versus fear; allow versus resist; tenderness versus tough; truth versus fear.
Trust in new physically stimulating journeys now. Believe it to be so.

Being a huge John Maher fan, I connected with various lyrics from repeated listening. One lyric epitomizes my post-crumble relations with running until recently, *"Can't wait to figure out what's wrong with me, so I can say this is the way I used to be, there's no substitute for time . . ."*

It's June 12th, an extremely warm, early summer is upon us. Reluctant perseverance gets me out for another walk/run interval routine down the lane at high noon. Tears stream down my cheeks, mixed in with salty sweat. To breathe properly is difficult as strong emotional heaves move through me with each step. My body craves the energy release running provides. Led Zeppelin's "Kashmir" blasts from my iPod, which fuels inner strength only ever felt when running, one that is addictive and empowering. I feel completely alive and in sync. This particular run sources my revelation to befriend uncertainty. More frequently, I pick up on vitalheart hits of sorts. Now, this is a high worthy of addiction. So, the message is, build trust in my body's ability to workout by respecting uncertainty instead of pushing it away in disdain.

I make a pact to commit to a physically active challenge to begin this fall. It is my way to utilize uncertainty to rise above fear and heal this trusting issue. In order for me to truly be landed in healing, I must overcome this fear of trust in my body's athletic ability.

> ♡ When you feel good, your emotional range would sweep from contentment to expectation, to eagerness, to joy. But, if you are giving your attention to the lack, or absence of your desire, your emotions would range from feelings of pessimism to worry to doubt to discouragement to anger, insecurity, depression—

> **this is the allowing creative process for each of us.**
> —*Ask and it is Given: Learning to Manifest Your Desires,* **by Esther and Jerry Hicks**

. . . .

A few weeks into nurturing my friendship with uncertainty, I witness a shift in how differently I approach things, in part due to a full reserve tank of strength and empowerment. Case in point is my annual pacemaker checkup. As my sweetie and I drive to the appointment, he says, *"You're controlling this experience, Chrissie,"* his way of encouraging me to determine how I will feel. I'm struck by his insight. An internal sense of certainty has landed for what I will insist upon during these appointments.

My *knowing* in childhood has come full circle. My non-negotiable is to leave the appointment if I'm not treated as a human being. I will no longer be subjected to the two tests that speed up and slow down my heartbeat—they will need to figure out another way so I'm comfortable and don't re-experience the ghastly feeling of passing out. I will not tolerate anything that reenacts and reinforces the initial trauma on a cellular level. I will no longer tolerate a clinical, detached approach or non-relationship with my heart's guardian, the doctor. I will not be rushed through my few questions to access their expertise—I'm a patient insisting on patience. I will no longer accept less than 100 percent respect and compassion.

This clarity is for me, but of equal importance for the next poor sod whose voice today is vulnerable, shaky and void of strength as was mine five years ago when I first landed in this office. It is a gesture to awaken an overly taxed system fatigued with lack of resources, complicated by a surplus of technology, and comatose to the power in the human touch. As long as I come to this office on an annual basis, I'll take it upon myself to define what acceptable human relations are when dealing with those in compromised states. In doing this, maybe the next person's family member will leave feeling a shred of empowerment to trust in their innate healing power ability.

When did current advancements in medical science and technology overshadow the extraordinary healing capacity of human touch, interaction and spirited encouragement? I sense that a reciprocal silence replacing emotional truth exists in many practitioner-patient relationships today. Patients possess innate knowing for what they may need, what *feels* right or not, and an educated sense to not automatically agree to the conventional prescription route. Media and access to information is playing a key role in this patient savvy that increasingly questions the Band-Aid concept, which diminishes resolve of core issues.

The independent, alternative modes of healing, which allow for co-directing a patient's dis-ease, are garnering respect and attention. The momentum is based on collectively defining the healing process, so individuals can tailor their own program. The astute patient will utilize a combination of the traditional, medical system practitioner guidance with complimentary, alternative ones to best determine an individualized plan of action. The wise choice: To lead in your own healing regime.

There is also the spiritual aspect of illness. By ignoring or denying illness in our lives through medicating only, we elude ourselves of the very message discomfort intends to deliver. How can we possibly appreciate vibrant health if we never experience its dark side, even if briefly? If aware, we can gain deep reverence for the duality of illness and vibrancy—whole health through navigating the dark side with our vitalheart guiding us.

There are many gifts that surface from our wounds. I am a testament to this. I've cultivated good relations with traditional and alternative practitioners and make it my business to initiate and maintain this process. The time has come for individuals to take responsibility for their health and not expect miracles from their practitioners if not taking care of their own temple. It's a two-way street.

So, back to the annual pacemaker checkup and the nurse's response to my non-negotiable. They stopped, heard and acted with compassion and respect. And, guess what? I soaked up my first neutral experience in that office in five years. I even scored a 10-minute one-on-one with the doctor, despite a waiting room full of ill-paced, fluttering hearts. Afterward, my sweetie reached over for my hand while driving the familiar roads and stated with much love, "*Watching you today with that smirk, seeing you glow, I realized . . . God, I really, really love her. I need to tell you this more often.*" When we choose to lead from authentic trust in truth, love responds in magical ways . . .

It remains my hope that I will eventually be completely healed on an energetic level from all that manifested my electrical short circuiting, my Heart*B*roke circumstances. When I no longer require this amazing gadget that currently keeps my heart paced, then I will have learned all intended for me. In the meantime, I'm humbly grateful for the unbelievable technology that bridges the gap between life and death for me.

♡ Creativity requires the courage to let go of certainties.
— Erich Fromm

* * * * * * * * * *

The IBS tummy challenges experienced the last two years can best be described as uncertain in terms of when it flares up. Last summer, this truly affected running, playing tennis and golfing. This year it is about 80 percent healed from plenty of trial-and-error research to heal the underlying cause.

My regimen includes: minimal dairy (organic); home-baked spelt and kamut bread products; no deep-fried foods; no beer; lots of greens; and good whole foods. In addition, I landed on Heather's Tummy website, which has been such a gift in supporting my system with peppermint oil capsules and acacia soluble fiber before each meal. The local vitamin store supplies me with digestive enzymes, acidophilus and aloe vera liquid. These work to keep the bacteria balanced in my gut and the liquid calms the irritated intestinal tract. As well, I was introduced to a series of hypnotic CDs that reprogram one's emotions on a cellular level—this vastly minimized many symptoms.

I can pretty much predict a tummy flare up with the consumption of mucho vino, the onset of my period or one too many desserts. This spring I have chosen to accept the uncertainty that my tummy reveals on some days. With a focus and detachment on complete resolve, I just went ahead and got active despite the discomfort. I've enjoyed golfing, tennis, seawall walks and lane runs while practicing trust that if it flares up, I'll be taken care of. I've played more golf this summer than the last five combined and cooled off on many scorching hot days with dips in the ocean.

Psychologically, I've known my tummy discomfort is stress based. Triggers are when my opinion isn't acknowledged when differing from those I'm close to—I don't need agreement, but do need a reciprocal desire to meet in the middle and respect for a difference in perspective. When I internalize truth to avoid the potential for conflict, it flares up; so, practicing courage in the moment instead of stuffing it down is essential.

Healing is a daily process with meditation, energetic medicine, yoga and awareness of self. I'm vigilant to take feelings of uncertainty and utilize them to nurture me from heart to tummy. Spiritually, I believe I created the IBS to protect myself from going out and pushing again. I have grown immensely from this uncertainty. It perfectly mirrors my need to befriend uncertainty once and for all. The time is near to give it permission to dissolve as I fully trust in my ability to live in balance and keep me safe. So, I will surrender it when the time is right for it to leave, knowing the time is close at heart.

Recently, an energetic body healer ended our session requesting I repeat *"it is safe to love my body."* I was overcome with a flood of tears. This energetic release ensued for a few minutes before I could choke out the words. The phrase is my latest mantra to recite as I increase physical activity.

Yes, a residual fear still exits, but I know resolve is inevitable in due course. In the meantime, I'm proud of the strides made with belief and practice in patience. I trust in what this period of time needs me to learn.

> An absolute can only be given in an intuition, while all the rest has to do with analysis.
> — Henri Bergson

Purpose and calling. I've come full circle in the entrepreneurial realm, which is amazing to me. Just a year ago, I didn't possess the trust to create another business vision. There was a lack of trust to maintain the lifestyle equilibrium created and cherished this past five years.

Without conscious recognition, the entrepreneur sneaked out of hiding. My love of writing jump-started things with a 30-day *Write the Damn Book* teleclass challenge after my business contract was terminated last winter. My thought was, if not now, then when, in terms of writing *the book*. It has been a humbling, revealing process and I'm tickled with the accomplishment of completing something I'm proud of.

At the same time, I pondered what is next for an income to carry me long term, productively and purposefully. I defined that my income needs to evolve as my expertise, wisdom and years do. I want a schedule that is flexible and revolves around my lifestyle, so I can give my best to self, family, friends and clients.

I want to be mobile and only require a laptop and telephone, doing my thing from anywhere on the planet. I want to build a practice that becomes richer in content and purpose with age—not age prohibited. Creative, passive, residual product income is a high priority. I want to witness utilizing my career and life experiences to date with absolute ease. That's it. Oh . . . and I want it to be fun, collaborative and rich in human exchange with like-minded souls. The exact nature and specifics of this income stream(s) is in the making and, for the first time in my adult life, I'm mostly at ease with letting it unfold. Each day, I cultivate www.healthmentorship.com—my new thing.

This health mentorship practice will provide a community where I can directly or indirectly inspire individuals toward optimum health for and with one another. I researched numerous educational programs and landed upon the e-Spirit program, an eight-month teleclass program I'm enrolled in . . . so, my horizons expand.

Unbeknownst to me for months, I now get that the book writing and entrepreneur spirit coaching program are complements to one another, creating the next vision. Time will tell how the vision unfolds.

The Law of Attraction premise is front and center in the e-Spirit coaching program. This premise holds close ties to the *trust in truth* premise. It's a no brainer to trust in abundance with unwavering belief when all is flowing. The real litmus test is seeing how I think, act and lead when things appear to be going sideways or backwards. My truth is revealed in all its naked charm in these moments, with much room to evolve ahead.

My current truth in relationship to abundance, or lack thereof, is this. When I participate with spirit, conviction and positivity, new sparks of progress toward my ideal just appear. When I disengage and participate with a half-assed attitude when things are not going as I planned, then my choices evaporate. If I only believe when all is swell and then abandon belief when fear appears, then I needn't expect anything too marvelous to land in my lap. So, I'm learning to practice grace with this notion in moments when fear needs to shift out of my consciousness.

> **You may be deceived if you trust too much, but you will live in torment if you don't trust enough.**
> — **Frank Crane**

Global uncertainty is at an all-time high. The associated fear of this pervades in the actions of most global leaders. The need to reflect on global consciousness, or lack thereof, is upon us. The opportunity to utilize the power of the individual heart and vitalheart voice to strengthen and heal the universal heart is on everyone's doorstep as conventional, worn-out ways force change as to what current truths are. The resulting shift in perspective lies in *possibilities* like no other period in modern civilization—to come together and reunite by trusting in the conscious, compassionate global heart. The spirit of this connection can override differences in religious, political or social beliefs if the notion of allowing various cultures to sort themselves out is acknowledged and adhered to.

To be successful, this needs to be permitted without attachment or conditions to the interim commercial and economic implications. This means that fear in all forms needs to bow down and surrender to the power of love. A Yin energy can balance the extremely Yang energy that has taken the world to its knees in the pursuit of greed, excess and unhealthy power and control.

Lack of understanding or denial that we are all connected, whether we like to admit it or not, is our biggest learning of all. With time, reflection and compassion, hopefully, we will witness a new way that is responsive versus reactive. This way may appear naïve or Pollyanna like to many. However, what I currently see is a sense of separateness and isolation, which is certainly not directing us down the path toward enlightenment—financially, socially or environmentally.

In casual conversations, most are hard pressed to hear another say they feel connected, secure and at ease. It's fascinating to wonder what individually and collectively will be created if we simply utilize the unprecedented advances in communication, technology, medicine, social and cultural acumen to complement moving us all forward with an open, trusting, compassionate and truthful heart.

There is much speculation of 2012 and what the implications are with the end of the Mayan calendar on December 21st. This date signifies a time of alignment of our planet, the solar system and center of our galaxy, which will not occur again for another 26,000 years. Witnessing and being apart of what can transpire as individuals evolve by choosing the conscious, collective heart route will be stunning. This influence can certainly bridge the gap of separateness presently felt globally. I believe the first step is in identifying what we are uncertain about and why from the mundane to the complex. Then, refreshed truths will lead our way.

> **You cannot solve any problem in the same state of consciousness in which it was created.**
> — Albert Einstein

. . . .

So, what's after this for me? I'm uncertain in a happy way, optimistic and quietly excited anyway!

As for my relationship with uncertainty—are we soul sisters yet? Here's *what is,* in signing off from these writings.

Grace. I intend to practice grace in uncertainty as my life evolves. I believe if I can master grace in uncertainty, then I may just be able to fulfill a productive purpose.

I'm choosing to shift my hardwired perspective with uncertainty. As my newly revered friend, she (uncertainty) will eventually symbolize an internal safety mechanism, one that I will respect, admire and cherish. She will gently alert my need for surrender to uncertain circumstances in order to trust uncovering a truth, thus transforming my potential.

The most profound losses, crises and upsets can take you to your knees. These same losses, crises and upsets can also transform expansion of spirit, character and heart to help others come through theirs. By helping others, the individual and collective global heart is genuinely enlightened through refined love, a love that stands for healing, hope and strength of character. The path of least resistance is certainly one way to go. However, the path of surrender, hope, tenacity and unity through uncertainty will no doubt conquer all not deemed good and consciously based. My biggest learning is this: If I trust in a truth, then transformation in self and for others always follows.

Soul sisters? Yes, we are now. Like any sisters, our days are a melting pot of laughter, reflection, struggle, support, healing and quiet empowerment inching forward. With trust, truth increases as love of heart and my vitalheart voice gently guide me along. As my friendship with uncertainty strengthens, my runs become a source of enjoyment, an opportunity to take in my surroundings. They are no longer runs away from unpleasant circumstances, but rather jogs gently guiding me toward new possibilities. We, me and my soul sister are becoming sufficient in the midst of possibilities and uncertainty. Living in a state of sufficiency is transformative.

> ♡ Uncertainty is the only certainty there is, and knowing how to live with insecurity is the only security.
> — John Allen Paulos

vitalheart tip Cultivate your ability to observe. You can learn more in five minutes of observation than by accessing information through questions. When you're consumed by the next question, you miss the subtle nuances, which speak volumes. You can resolve your disquiet with observation. Try feeling your way through an interaction by utilizing your vitalheart voice instead of your mind—notice the revelations.

connect possibilities
body · mind · spirit · heart

INTERNET RESEARCH

Abraham Hicks . . . . www.lawofattractioninteraction.com

Deeksha Blessing . . . . www.onenessuniversity.com

Eknath Easwaran . . . . www.easwaran.org

Gary Renard . . . . www.garyrenard.com

Gwenyth Paltrow's GOOP. . . . . www.goop.com

Heal Your Life . . . . www.healyourlife.com

Online Publisher. . . . . www.outskirts.com

Spiritualpreneur Coaching Program. . . . .
www.e-spiritcoaching.com

Step-Parenting . . . . www.blendedfamiles.com

Brain Sync . . . . www.brainsync.com

DO

Energetic Body Healing . . . . www.bodytalksystems.com

Tracy Anderson Workout . . . www.tracyandersonmethod.com

www.healthmentorship.com

If you enjoyed reading my book, you will certainly benefit from www.healthmentorship.com.

The online experience intends to utilize a collective strength of expertise, experience and fun to inspire and provoke you to shift thoughts into action by trusting in truth. The vitalheart voice—your intuition—is the base tool cultivated to do just this!

Shared resources, tools, and perspectives will encourage your shift with uncertainty from fear to fabulousness by getting real on a given truth. The more you tap into truth, the greater potential lived—emotionally, spiritually, financially, physically and intellectually. If uncertainty is zapping your sense of ease, self and humor out of the daily experience, you need to reclaim it. Once again, feel your presence by creating new possibilities from the most troublesome circumstances.

Conveniently, this is all at your fingertips or headset without leaving the comfort of home or office. Uncertainty can become your greatest pal, gifting insights to the next best thing coming your way.

Visit www.healthmentorship.com

- Get inspired—receive the complimentary quarterly *Trust in Truth* e-newsletter

- Enroll in the *From Uncertainty to Fabulousness* webinar programs

- Access international presenters, everyday tools and products with bonus gifts

- Learn about our telephone *Marketing Mentor* program for entrepreneurs and small business owners to create a vision for a lifestyle first, career second

- Enroll in the monthly *Business Collaborator* webinars

**TO RECEIVE MY COMPLIMENTARY GIFT,
SIMPLY REGISTER AT
HTTP:// BOOKPROMO.HEALTHMENTORSHIP.COM**

To customize a webinar program or
book speaking engagements,
call (604) 347-5990.
www.healthmentorship.com
christine@healthmentorship.com

give-back and collaborative partners

As I wrote this book and created www.healthmentorship.com, I decided that giving back and collaboration are two business non-negotiables.

For me, giving back is about extending my message to influence and complement another's like-minded approach, to somehow assist in enhancing their purpose. The idea of creating a book club fund where book club goers leave with a brand new book in hand after connecting with the author or book-related expert is right up my alley. I LOVE books! I've always loved: their individual look, feel and smell; the anticipation of where the words will take me as I carry it home from the bookstore; the visual I create within as I associate with the characters; various perspectives that challenge my own; the power and magic of an author's imagination; passing a terrific read on to a friend because they have to read it; the notion that books are individuals in the form of words. I LOVE books, so $1 from each book sold will be donated to a book club fund for Dress for Success Vancouver.

Collaboration is pragmatic, effortless, fun and profitable. My overall business model philosophy is to live a desired lifestyle with a career built around it. This means efficiency, discipline and clarity in terms of time management, energy expended and overall marketing cohesiveness. Like-minded and complementary connections come to mind describing collaborative partners. My intent is to provide value to my partners through my marketing promotions while delivering exceptional, unique offerings to you, the reader, webinar participant, marketing mentor client.

GIVE-BACK PARTNER

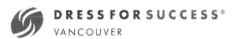

One dollar from each book sold will go toward establishing and operating a facilitated Book Club, free to Dress for Success Vancouver clients. The intent is by reading and then coming together to discuss ideas, which the book(s) generate, clients will have the opportunity to communicate openly, and listen to and absorb diverse perspectives. The Book Club will help establish habits of learning, communication and respect for alternate opinions; habits that, in turn, contribute to a woman's success in the workplace.

At **Dress for Success Vancouver**, we believe that every woman, regardless of her financial circumstances, has the ability to succeed. To that end, we assist low-income women by providing not only working wardrobes, but also support services that will allow them to transition into the workforce and progress towards self-sufficiency. Our Mission is to promote the economic independence of economically disadvantaged women by providing professional attire, a network of support and the career development tools to help women thrive in work and in life. www.dressforsuccess.org/vancouver

COLLABORATIVE PARTNERS

ALLImax Canada	www.allimax.ca
Alycia Hall	www.alyciahall.com
Brita McLaughlin Coaching	www.britamclaughlincoaching.com
Chatelaine Magazine	www.chatelaine.com
Coaching From Spirit Institute	www.coachingfromspirit.com
Dress for Success Vancouver	www.dressforsuccess.org/vancouver
Grace Cirocco Inc	www.gracecirocco.com
NGNG Enterprises (No Guts No Glory)	www.insightfulDevelopment.com
Nutrition House	www.nutritionhouse.com
Preferred Nutrition	www.pno.ca
Sally Shields	www.thedilrules.com
Vivvos Fashion	www.vivvos.com

Made in the USA
Charleston, SC
04 November 2010